# So You Have Heart Disease So Do We

## Linda J. Phillips, R.N.

**Writers Club Press**
San Jose · New York · Lincoln · Shanghai

**So You Have Heart Disease...So Do We**

Published by Writers Club Press
an imprint of iUniverse.com, Inc.

For information address:
iUniverse.com, Inc.
620 North 48th Street
Suite 201
Lincoln, NE 68504-3467
www.iuniverse.com

This book is not intended to be a medical guide. The experiences related are
the express true experiences of the contributors in this book. It is in no way
is to be used in substitution for medical advise by any person.

ISBN: 0-595-09594-1

Printed in the United States of America

*I dedicate this book with all my love to my husband and children, whose love and devotion to me will always be treasured.*

*To the memory of the woman who inspired me to live my life, my Mother, the most gracious lady I have ever known—*

*Berma Landrum.*

# Contents

**Introduction: Divine Healing**                                    237

**Divine Experience Contributors: Divine Healing/Miracle:**

# Preface

A divinely inspired book for the support of heart patients, by heart patients.

Heart patients share their personal experiences with you to offer you encouragement from their real life experiences.

You are your own best caregiver. These patients show you how to obtain the best that medical technology has to offer in the treatment of Cardiovascular Disease.

You will also find angel encounters as told by the people that experienced them. You will learn how these experiences changed their lives for the better, and how they felt God's presence surrounding them.

You will explore healing miracles revealed by personal testimony of the people that witnessed or experienced divine healing themselves.

# Acknowledgments

The first and foremost acknowledgment I would like to make is to the real author of this book—the Holy Spirit. The divine inspiration to author this book became a driving force in my life.

I wish to give special thanks to my husband, Stan, for keeping me in focus while undertaking this divine endeavor. He was a balancing factor in keeping me on track from its inception. He constantly encouraged me to go forward with what God told me to do.

The support and love shown to me by my children, Allen and Brigette, gave me the inspiration to go higher in my endeavors. When I questioned my ability to accomplish my goal, I heard "Mom you can do it." That inspired me to proceed.

Thank you to the wonderful people that shared their heart disease experiences with me. These experiences will give encouragement and support to others with heart disease, their families and friends. The overwhelming response and encouragement from them indicated that I was on the right track and following God's direction to help others. Without the time and talents of the participants who contributed their stories, this book would not be a reality. May God bless each of them in their individual circumstances in life.

I would like to give special thanks to Misty Craddock for her support and help with heart patient research and encouraging these heart patients to participate in this project. Misty is an informed source on the latest in research into the new techniques and treatment for heart patients; and she always shared her knowledge and research.

Where would my life be without the influence of Brother Gordon Dacre? He is the backbone of my spiritual guidance. His encouragement and discernment on my life according to will of God is an unfailing constant support to me.

My special thanks goes to my wonderful friend of a lifetime Johnnie Mae Keyes, who would patiently allow me to share my ideas, grumble, and laugh during the long months spent developing this project.

The credit for editing goes to Christine Brown. Her expertise and guidance is greatly appreciated. Thank you, Christine, for your patience and understanding with me.

# Introduction:
# Heart Disease Experiences

God is AWESOME.

I have lived with a catastrophic disease for the last seven years.

This book is written because medical professionals forget to tell heart patients about the emotional aspects of heart disease. It is intended to provide support for all heart patients, no matter what their specific diagnosis may be. If you are a heart patient, this book can help you better understand the physical and emotional changes you experience from heart disease. If your heart is the problem, then this book is for you.

Heart disease remains the number one killer of men and women. Medical strides for the improvement of treatment has advanced rapidly in the past ten years. My main qualification for writing this book is that it was given to me by divine inspiration to help heart patients with the support of heart patients. You will not find complicated medical jargon in this book. I am a Registered Nurse and have now experienced this disease as a caregiver and as a patient. This disease can be devastating, which is why this book is specifically dedicated to heart patients. I do know from my personal experience something emotional changes when it is your heart that is affected. It can't be clearly explained, but I do know that a change happens. Doctors do not get into the emotional aspects of this disease on a routine basis. The emotional trauma is as devastating as the physical illness. Some patients are able to work their way through the emotional crisis, yet some are not.

The emotional acceptance of a diagnosis of heart disease, as you will see in this book, sometimes does not come easy. Many times the diagnosis of heart disease is overlooked because the patients do not express typical symptoms. This statement is especially true for women. Women with symptoms of heart disease are often overlooked unless the doctor is fine-tuned to detecting symptoms specific to women. Medical facts show that symptoms in women are atypical from the gripping chest pain and shortness of breath reported by men. Often this can lead to a disastrous ending for women. Heart disease was once thought to be a disease of growing old, unless you were born with a birth defect. Now, as you will see in the following pages, that heart disease is not an exclusive illness of the elderly. If you presented yourself at the age of 30 with chest pain in your doctor's office, nine times out of ten you would be told, "You're under to much stress, cut down on your caffeine," and sent on your merry way. This creates confusion, and often you are left wondering "What does it take for me to know what is physically wrong with me?"

The answer...be as informed as you can. Get involved in your medical care. Push! Remember you won't make friends all the time, but you will get results! Sometimes I think patients like myself try to diagnose instead of being informed, and placate over needs rather than demand that your care is the best that it can be. After all, you are not trying to make life long friends that will send you flowers if you won't be around to enjoy them.

Even with the vast improvements in the technology of diagnostics, medications and advanced life saving procedures, heart disease remains the number one killer in our society. Why? We are told to cut down on fats, watch your cholesterol, lose weight, exercise, and lower your stress. Certainly we should try to maintain a healthy life style, in addition to ensuring our bodies are active physically and mentally. DON'T SMOKE! That is one of the largest factors in maintaining a healthy heart. Haven't you heard this terrible scenario before? "George dropped dead from a heart attack." George didn't smoke, ate healthy, and ran five miles a day. He stayed at a perfect weight, had an annual physical, and had no problems with his cholesterol or triglycrides, yet he died from a heart attack. Doesn't this make you wonder what a person can control when it comes to health? You live your life doing all the things your doctor tells you to do, you sacrifice some of the finer things in life to be healthy, and the next thing you know you're having bypass surgery.

Don't get me wrong, the medical profession, of which I have been proud to be a part of for 22 years, is a wonderful profession. I dedicated my life-long vocation to medicine. But, medicine is not an exact science. As you will come to realize by the time you finish this book, there are elements in this world that are beyond our control or understanding. We do all the "right" things and the "right things" are not enough.

The subject of women and heart disease has come to the forefront in the past 15 years. When women with heart disease were treated, they usually died. Men were easily diagnosed, and women were not. If women lived around large medical centers, they had an increased chance to receive better treatment. Doctors considered heart disease as a man's disease. One of the largest factors affecting heart disease in men was and is stress. Back then, women were usually homemakers. This was not viewed as a stressful occupation by the medical profession. With the women's movement that started in 1960's, women traded their aprons in for business suits. Women's health issues gained attention because they had better access to health care.

Heart disease, no matter what gender it affects, manifests as a physically and emotionally devastating disease. The common dominator according to heart patients is FEAR. In many instances heart attacks can strike without warning. One day you're looking forward to a bright future, and then, in an instant you are left to wonder if you will have a future at all. Doctors may treat the physical side of you, but neglect the emotional side of this disease. On the inside you question your sanity and the outlook for your future. Little has been said about the powerful emotions that follow an episode with the heart, or the thoughts and emotions that stem from living with a chronic form of the disease. The diagnosis of heart disease is for life. Many patients can experience a denial stage; they refuse to accept that anything happened to them. But, once a heart patient, always a heart patient. Strength is a characteristic of the human species. If we reveal our feelings we are afraid of being labeled "weak" or, labeled as a person preoccupied with health.

As I mentioned earlier, something happens to you when your heart is involved. Ask any heart patient how they felt emotionally after a heart attack. Reluctant to talk about it, afraid that they are alone with their feelings, only to find out that they are not. While researching the stories for this book, I was overwhelmed with the response after contacting these heart patients. To the participants and contributors, thank you for doing this project. Most of the heart patients I spoke with or read their experience felt that they would rather talk with another heart patient than with their medical professional. A fellow heart patient is someone that understands what heart patients are experiencing and is more important than medical jargon.

After all, if your heart doesn't beat the next beat, where does that leave you? Heart disease has a way of chasing you night and day with your own mortality. Many say they have "night terrors." They are afraid to go to sleep, or are afraid they will wake up during the night with something wrong. Many patients fear the "heart attack" mode the hospital emergency room staff goes into if you come to the hospital and present yourself with symptoms. Most heart patients experience fear in traveling to any location that is a significant distance from available medical care. They wonder if it will happen because it has already happened once before without warning. Patients that experience chest pain on a regular basis express the fear that "Will my medicine make it go away or is this the one that won't go away?" Many patients that have near death episodes with heart disease live with post-traumatic stress syndrome, much like Vietnam veterans returning to the U.S. after the war.

There is hope. Medical technology advances are discovered daily for the treatment of this catastrophic disease. This book is an open, honest account. At times it may seem depressing. It is not meant to be. The intention is to inform the newly diagnosed heart patient of the unspoken effects they may experience, as well as, give support to patients with chronic heart disease. Patients, families and friends need this information, because a lack of understanding of heart disease and its effects is the basis for most of the fears heart patients' experience. We fear the unknown and most of us lack someone to talk to that we feel will understand. My intention is to let this book be a support mechanism to help alleviate fears of the heart patient or a family member that will read this book. Your doctor usually will not discuss with you the emotional side of heart disease, because most have not experienced that side of the heart disease. Experience is the best teacher and most heart patients are willing and eager to lend an ear in support of each other. Find a heart buddy and fight the good fight against heart disease. It is not all gloom and doom. God in his infinite wisdom will show you the way and ease your fears. Before you go to bed, give all your fears to him, after all, He will be up all night anyway. He has been there for me and He will be there for you.

I am a firm believer that genetics play a large role in helping to find the answers to some of the "Why?" questions. God created this masterpiece of a body and fine-tuned it like a harp. But, down through the centuries, man played a major role in tipping the scales of the human body out of balance. We, as heart patients can stand together and hopefully realign the balance. We need to take care of ourselves to the best of our ability, follow our doctor's advice, get involved, and don't be afraid to ask for a second opinion. Any doctor that objects to you seeking the advice of another medical professional may have a lack of confidence in his/her ability to diagnose. If you encounter this situation, move on. It's your life—no one can live it but you.

God created a unique individual in each of us and our experiences are our own. Do all you can do and then stand in faith. As the saying goes, bad things do happen to good people. We have seen this through centuries past and will see this in centuries to come. Be a survivor, not a victim.

I hope these collective experiences enlightened you so you will feel comfortable with what to expect in your progress combating heart disease. The experiences, you will read were written by the heart patients themselves. I have not altered them in any way. The experiences appear exactly as each author wanted to relate them to you. Please keep in mind that we are all different emotionally and physically. Our ability to cope with each individual circumstance is up to us.

*Steve's story shows us that he is an inspiration to all of us. His message not only deals with heart disease, but also touches the essence of our existence to fight to live life to it's fullest.*

*Hebrews 11:1 "Now faith is the substance of things hoped for, the evidence of things not seen."*

# "10 Years of Agony"
## By
## Steve

As a heart patient, my life changed dramatically about 10 years ago. I knew my family on both sides had a history of heart problems, but being in the prime of my life, I didn't give the family history a second thought. At least 2 generations back all had cardiac related disease and at least half of my family died from heart attacks way before their time.

But, I was only in my 40s, and nothing could happen to me. Then, one winter day, I suddenly started to feel a sharp, hot burning pain in the center of my chest. It scared the living daylights out of me. It slowly radiated from the center of my chest toward my shoulders. I didn't want to think about the cause, I simply wanted to get relief, treatment, or tell it to go away on its own. It didn't. I was at work, then. The first thing I did was call my wife, and tell her to leave her job early, right then, and come pick me up and get me to the hospital emergency room. My doctor's offices were at least another half-hour away from the hospital —it seemed at the time the quickest way to get treatment. As it turned out, it was the wisest decision I have ever made. Within one to two hours of the onset of the pain and burning, I was being treated for a major MI at the hospital with TPA and other 'wonder' medications. After getting me stabilized and doing some preliminary tests and treatments, the cardiologist decided I needed further 'work'—and that amounted to a trip to another hospital for a TCPA (Balloon Angioplasty). The doctors at this particular hospital didn't have the staff or the equipment to handle it there. From the onset of the pain, my mind was numb. I didn't want to think about the consequences. I didn't want to even admit that I was now becoming a heart patient. I didn't want to think about 'diminished capacity,' or any change in my lifestyle. I was a hard worker, and I was working six and seven days a week. I had my own optical practice. I had a wife (and she had 2 growing children). I had numerous other obligations, which required my attention every day of every week. What was going to happen to all this? How was I going to handle them? Where would I wind up after 'all the dust settled' and what kind of condition would I have been in?

It was a living nightmare. It was hell experienced first-hand. To make matters even worse, it was Christmas of 1989. Not a time to be in a hospital bed, alone with all those fears and thoughts, too much time to think and not enough physical ability to do much else. My mind was numb. I was angry. Angry with myself, angry with my body betraying me, and angry with everyone for every little thing that wasn't going right in my life. Anger took over the thought processes. One night during my hospitalization, I was so angry that I woke up in the middle of the night and pulled out all my wires and plugs from the various machines and monitors that were serving to ease the strain on my heart. I started to get out of bed before I was even awake enough to realize what I was doing. That was the beginning of 10 years of agony, fears, and anger. After leaving the hospital, the Cardiologist put me in a Rehab program. The program gave me back my physical stamina, but did not erase the psychological scars. I was a different person. I was angry, scared, and defiant.

In 1992, after 2 years of returning to physical 'normalcy,' I suddenly experienced a 2nd M. I. During those 2 years, I was working and trying to lead a 'normal' life, tending to my obligations, making a living, but still under that psychological cloud of anger and fear. It affected everything I did. When I was rushed to the hospital with the 2nd heart attack, and then transported to another hospital for a quadruple C.A.B.G., it was another, even more serious blow to my ego, psyche, and self-esteem. My marriage was rocky, my ability to work was diminished, my ability to function was hampered, and I still had all of the same responsibilities and obligations. Living became even more difficult. My heart was now functioning at about half its normal level. I became tired easily, more irritated quickly.

I functioned on an 'existence' level. Former pleasures were no longer enjoyable.

In 1994, the Mitral Valve gave out, and I wound up in the hospital for a third major procedure. This one took eleven hours to complete because of all the scar tissue. As you can well imagine, it did nothing to make living easier. Fear, anger and defiance became a way of life. My heart was now working at about forty percent of its normal level, and I was now living with a steady, constant 'ticking' sound that was audible to those around me in a quiet room. I felt like a time bomb, ticking away, waiting for some unknown hand to push the 'detonate' button. I was not strong enough to work any longer, and went on long-term disability. This became a way of life that has existed until recently.

During the last five to six years, I have been in the hospital several times with congestive heart failure, treated for pneumonia, and have had to lead a more sedentary life style. I have had to find the level of activity that my body can safely handle, even though my mind wants to do a hundred things more. I tire more quickly. I anger more quickly. I am on thirteen different medications and three inhalers. I have been in the hospital recently for another TCPA with stent. I have had, in short, so many changes in my life that I have made many adjustments. At one point, a couple of years ago, I decided that I had enough of feeling sorry for myself and I decided to make a change in my goals.

I went back to school for a degree in computers, even though I already had a profession. Since I didn't have the stamina to do my former profession, I reasoned it was time to set some new goals and look to a profession that I might be able to handle. Ticking away, I went back to school. I also decided to try my hand at a part-time job, to see if I could handle the physical demands, and to help out financially in the family setting. Changing my outlook, even with the new goals and added physical demand of a job, has been, and still continues to be, the hardest job I have ever done in my life. Improving my self-esteem, raising my level of patience, setting realistic goals and learning to live within those guidelines is, and will continue to be, a way of life that will demand the utmost of me.

But I'm a fighter. I'm not going to go passively. I am going to kick and battle my way every day until the end. I'm going to use the experiences and lessons of the past years to, as the US Army ad says, 'be all that I can be.' I believe that the Good Lord has some plan for me, and I do not intend to sit idly by and let the 'parade pass me by'. I am as active as I can be, given what I have to work with, and will continue to work on the weak spots. Sitting in a rocking chair waiting for the 'grim reaper' is not my idea of life. Yes, life is much, much different now than ten years ago, but those lessons and the battles fought will make me a stronger person. I hope that this little biographical sketch will help others come to realize that there is 'life after a heart attack', and will adjust their lifestyles accordingly. We are not the same people we were before, and that does not mean that we are less. We are just different. Those around us must learn patience with us, as we must with ourselves. We must learn to deal with our anger, feelings of depression and helplessness, diminished capacities, and health issues as a challenge; just another of life's opportunities to achieve a new goal and learn a new lesson. Each day is another opportunity to help others in our situation, learn something new and different, be and act according to the golden rule, and enjoy life and the wonders and happiness around us. I'm learning that lesson every day.

Steve Rosenthal

Mended Hearts Chapter 244, Cocoa Beach FLA.

VP Space Coast P. C. Users Group, also of Cocoa FLA.

*I would like to thank you Judy for sharing your uplifting experience with us.*

# My New Beginning

My name is Judy Kenniston and I was born with a deformed Aortic Valve. But I wasn't aware of it until I was 21 and the doctor told me I had a heart murmur. It didn't seem important then because heart murmurs are so common.

However, at the age of 46, during my annual physical, my doctor told me my murmur was very loud and I was referred to a Cardiologist who performed an echocardiogram. The next morning I received a call from his office saying I needed to return. That was the beginning of a frightening whirlwind for me. I had been diagnosed with severe Aortic Stenosis. Which means severe narrowing of the valve. A normal valve's opening is approx. 2.5 cm and mine was .47cm.

When the doctor told my husband and me the news, we sat there shocked. How could this be happening to me? I'm young, healthy and asymptomic. That's when my husband asked the doctor how accurate the test was. He said, very accurate and he would 'bet the farm on it'. My husband saw a picture of him standing proudly beside his sailboat so he asked "but would you bet your boat?" He leaned back in his chair, smiled and said, "I'd bet the boat." That's when I knew I was in trouble.

The Cardiologist told us that I had 2 choices:

1. Watchful Waiting

(Which entailed waiting for a symptom and then replacing the valve)

He explained the symptom as Sudden Death. I never did understand how that could be a symptom.

OR

2. Replace the Valve.

I told the doctor that I believed in preventative maintenance. And if my fan belt were cracked I wouldn't wait to break down on the side of the road before replacing it.

Then he explained my three choices for replacement.

1. Replace my valve with a Pig's valve (which lasts approximately 10 yrs.)

2. Replace it with a mechanical valve (and live on blood thinners like Coumidin).

Or

3. Do what they call the "Ross Procedure." This procedure was first done by Dr. Ross in England in 1967 but wasn't accepted in the states until the late 1980s. It's where they take your Aortic Valve off and replace it with your Pulmonary Valve. Then they get a human donor's Pulmonary Valve to replace yours.

Well, this was a no brainer for me. I opted for the Ross Procedure. But my doctor explained that you have to qualify for this surgery. He said you have to be less than 50 years old, very healthy with no cholesterol problems or bypass surgery needed. Be active enough to not want to take blood thinners because of the bleeding risks involved. Luckily, I qualified, and received the Ross Procedure on October 28, 1998. And now, here I am, fully healed and able to do more physically than I've done in years.

I feel very fortunate for several reasons. Not only have I been given a second chance in life, but also now I'm able to truly see things in a way I couldn't before. I'm the lucky one.

I remember when I was lying on the surgery table getting my heart catherization before my surgery. My cardiologist saw how bad my valve was and said "Judy, I know you were hoping for good news, and wanted to be able to wait five to ten years, but its pretty bad and we need to fix it now." I started to cry and said, " Its not that I mind having surgery, it's the fact that I'm broken. I feel like I've been marked down by the cardiologist and put on the Sale Rack—Imperfect". He smiled and said "Gee, no one has ever said that to me before." I guess we all go through life thinking we are healthy and invincible, then all of a sudden we are faced with this mortality issue. It was hard for me to sit in the cardiologist office looking at all the patients over 65 years old. I didn't feel like I belonged there. I wasn't ready for heart problems I wasn't old enough to be sick.

Then after the surgery I dealt with the fear of thinking, "Can it happen again?" Every little twinge scared me. I would wake up at night having panic attacks until I was able to go through Cardiac Rehab, which gave me the confidence of being able to physically function without fear.

I'm also dealing with my scar issue. My scar didn't heal well and both physically and emotionally, and it's been difficult. After much prompting by my family and friends to "wear it as a medal." I allowed it to show on a few occasions and had people either cringe at the sight, whisper to other people to look, and at one time actually had a girl jump back and say "Geeze, its going to get better right?" Well, after having tears well up too many times, I've decided to go to a Dermatologist for Cortisone injections, which should at least flatten my scar, and hopefully, have it turn white like a stretch mark. I should start treatment February 2.

But the most difficult part of this experience is the sadness it has caused me. I think of what has happened and just cry. But on the other hand, I feel lucky to have had this opportunity to re-evaluate my life. I remember thinking before my surgery. If today is my last day can I say I have lived well? And the answer was "No, you could have done better." But now God has given me the opportunity to change some things and do a better job with the time I have left. Not everyone has been given an "eye-opening" awareness like me. So I feel like I'm the lucky one.

*Larry's uplifting story helps to balance the scales of heart disease patients. As you hear his positive attitude, you will see that it reflects his eagerness to cope, to fight the battle and always strive to come out on the other side. This is the goal of all heart patients and with a strong faith, determined attitude, the support of a loving family even the smallest step is a victory.*

# Larry's Heart Experience

I had a major MI at age 48, got to the hospital soon enough to have TPA administered which worked to avoid major heart muscle damage. I ended up with some muscle damage but nothing that couldn't be worked with. I was transferred to another hospital where I had the catherization (angioplasty). I remained in the hospital a few days and then went home. I started cardiac rehab about six weeks after the MI and completed a twelve week monitored program. I continued in a phase four rehab program at a local fitness club and did very well with exercise, weight loss, and lowering of cholesterol and trigylcerides. I went a total of eleven months and had a second MI. I was able to recognize the symptoms soon enough to get to the hospital and avoid more heart damage. The catherization was done, and they decided this was obviously not a fluke, so bypass surgery was indicated. I had an uneventful surgery (three hours start to finish) and was off the respirator by 4:15 p.m., and awake again at 7:00 p.m. I stayed awake all night bugging the SICU nursing staff for food! My recovery was pretty uneventful also, with the exception of an episode of atrial fibrillation which was treated with medication IV, and then 3 doses of oral medicine after the IV was completed. I attended an expedited but abbreviated cardiac rehab program again and then returned to my health club. I control my weight, cholesterol, triglycerides and now my adult onset diabetes with medication, diet, and intense exercise. I have moved my exercise levels up to super step aerobics and cardio kickboxing. I now exercise at 10 to 11 MET level, which equals to work task of heavy construction or lumbering. I am so busy and feel so good that it is hard to believe where I've been over the last three years. As a matter of fact, most medical people have a hard time believing that I've been through all this since as they say "You don't look as if you've ever had a sick day in your life." This is not to say that there haven't been emotional issues involved, or my share of down days, but I have been very fortunate to have uncounted numbers of people supporting and encouraging me which I help credit my progress. Last year I won one of 20 honorable mentions in the "Ecotrin Heart Patient of the Year" award program and have a better than average chance of winning the award for 1999.

Larry Walker

*Women with heart disease have come to the forefront at an alarming rate. Awareness of women's issues in heart disease has shown that it can attack at any age.*

# Heart Disease: My Story
## By
## Carol

Family History: My paternal grandfather died at the age of 46 from a massive heart attack. My father had his first heart attack at the age of 38 and his second six months later. One of his brothers died at the age of 44 from a massive heart attack. Also one of my mother's brothers died at the age of 44 of a massive heart attack.

At the age of 33, I started having tightening in my chest and it went up into my neck. It felt like when you have the flu and your body aches. It was just in my neck and chest area. I also had a lot of indigestion and heartburn and thought at that time that it might be indigestion that was causing the problem. But family members insisted I see my doctor, so I did. I was then given medication for the indigestion and heartburn. The medication took care of the indigestion and heartburn, but I was still having the tightening and aches, especially when I was at work. I went back for my follow up appointment and told my doctor I was still having the tightening. He then sent me to have a stress test where they injected dye into my arteries and then took pictures of my heart. The test showed that blood was not passing through my arteries the way it should have.

My doctor then sent me to a specialist in Burlington, Vermont, where I received excellent care. I had a catherization done and found that I had one artery eighty percent blocked and one that was one hundred percent blocked.

At that time I was given the option of having bypass surgery or having stent placement done. I chose to have stent placement done because my father had stent placement done and he is doing well. I had a stent placed in the artery that was eighty percent blocked in December of 1997. I went back in January of 1998 to have a stent placed in the artery that was one hundred blocked, but were unable to open the blockage.

I was a smoker, but quit in December when I found out I had heart disease. I worried a lot about not having a full life and was afraid when I go to sleep that I won't wake up. I realized that worrying all the time would not help matters—it will only make things worse. I still have tightening when my medication wears off. But for the most part, I am doing well.

I have other health problems to deal with I have Menieres disease and also presumed Ocular Histoplasmosis Sydrome along with heart disease. I deal with them the same way. I just try not to let it bother me. It's very hard, but its something I have to deal with.

Carol Love
Age 35
Northern New York

*Susan shares her diagnosis and treatment of this rare cardiac condition.*

*"And Jesus saith unto him, I will come and Heal him."*
*Matthew 8:7*

# Prinzmetal's Angina

Hello!

I have a rare condition called Prinzmetal's Angina. Please feel free to use my story.

Seven years ago, I was awakened because of severe pain in my chest or stomach.

I had no idea about the origin or cause of the pain. All I knew was that if I took a slug of Mylanta; the pain would shortly disappear. Although I was sweating profusely and had pain radiating down my left arm, the pain went away in about five minutes. After this experience occurred several times during the night, I asked a pharmacist whether or not he thought I had heartburn. He insisted that I visit my doctor immediately. The doctor first chose to check my heart and referred me to a cardiologist. I had an EKG (normal) and all the stress tests (normal). The cardiologist then referred me to a gastroenterologist. I had an upper GI and endoscopy. The upper GI indicated that I had severe GERD and a hiatus hernia. The Endoscopy indicated that my esophagus and stomach were normal. The gastroenterologist immediately prescribed Zantac, but he also prescribed Nitroglycerin for severe attacks. I thought I was finally going to get a good night sleep when I took the first Zantac.

Wrong! I was wakened again by the same pain, so I took the Nitro. The pain quickly went away. I called the gastroenterologist the next day to tell him what had happened.

Because I have dystonia, he thought I was having spasms of my esophagus. Before having me undergo a test even he thought was terrible, he suggested that I wear a Holter monitor for 24 hours. During this time, I had four episodes of pain. The cardiologist called my office and told me to come to the office—ASAP.

Needless to say, I was frightened. The monitor showed abnormalities each time I recorded a pain episode.

The cardiologist told me that I might have something called Prinzmetal's Angina. This problem is sometimes called unstable angina. The coronary arteries go into spasm. With the usual angina, this would show up during a stress test. With Prinzmetal's, the spasms typically occur when the heart is at rest. I had a coronary catherization and had an episode on the operating table. The films showed that the arteries in my left ventricle were completely closed. It was kind of funny, in retrospect. The illness is rare and is almost never caught during an angiogram.

We first tried Nitro patches, but I was allergic to the adhesive. Then we tried a calcium channel blocker. The common drugs did not do the job. The last drug I tried, Verelan worked.

In short (or long), that is my story. The cause of this condition is unknown. I had surgery on my right sternocleidomastoid muscle several years ago, due to the dystonia, so there is some thought that the vagus nerve was affected.

Susan Becraft

*God in his infinite wisdom always has an answer for his children.
"Beloved, I wish above all things that thou mayest prosper and be
in health, even as thy soul prospereth."
3 John 2*

# Mary Arehart's Heart Experience

11 November 1999

Not exactly sure where to begin so I will go back to the very beginning. In December of 1992 I married the man of my dreams. He and I were old friends and I hadn't seen him for ten years when we got back together.

I have a 14 year old, son from a previous relationship and had been a single mother all his life. Jeremy, my son, and Nick, my husband got along wonderfully and I felt truly blessed. In January of 1994 we decided to have a child and I was amazed how easily I got pregnant. We spent most of 1994 getting ready for our new baby boy and we found a lovely house in a really nice neighborhood just short of our baby's birth in November.

Well, things were wonderful even though I had had a tough pregnancy and my delivery turned into an emergency C-section. I had been put on medical leave because my blood pressure was so high and my swelling pretty severe. Looking back, now I know that the baby was hard on my already "in-trouble" heart. I went back to work the following January in 1995. I was an Administrative Assistant for Orkin Exterminating Companies North Georgia Region office and my job was an extremely hectic and stressful one, but I always thought that I thrived on stress and loved the job. I had started with them as a bookkeeper in Clearwater, Florida, and worked my way up pretty quickly because of my ability to "get it done."

I started missing a lot of work, feeling really poorly but not being able to really explain my symptoms. By June of 1995, I was having terrible pain in my jaw and throat that would come and go and pain in my ears. I went to my family doctor, and he decided I had TMJ. He gave me some kind of muscle relaxant and sent me home. One night I woke up with the most incredible pain in my throat that I have ever experienced and then it went away. I went to work the next day driving down to our Newnan branch to check on things. I started feeling pretty bad and weak and decided to go home and the whole trip home my jaw was killing me. That night about 10:00 p.m., the pain in my jaw became so severe that I was crying hysterically and telling my husband that I needed to go to the emergency room. Before I could get dressed the pain had worked its way into my face and I could feel it crawling through every nerve.

At the hospital I was fortunate that they immediately started me on Nitro IV and the next day did a stress test. When he came in my room and told me that I did indeed have a heart attack (non q-wave) and that he was going to do a cardiac catherization right then, I was stunned. This couldn't be happening. Here I was with a new baby, a son in his teens and a new husband. Surely God wasn't going to take that all away from me now! The catherization showed that I had two arteries: one sixty percent blocked, the other ninety five percent blocked, and they were whisking me away to another hospital to perform angioplasty with stents on both of the arteries, left coronary and right coronary. The operation came before I had time to absorb all of this. Before I knew it, I was back home. I was in shock and my mom and sister had come up to help my husband, children and me. Now, I had been a smoker since I was about thirteen. My father had died of CAD at age 62, although it was never diagnosed because he would not ever go to a doctor. I spent the next few weeks in a total fog scared to move or breathe.

Every little pain scared the hell out of me and I just constantly cried. I had a bottle of Fiorinal I had been taking for really bad headaches and I was eating them as if it were candy, keeping myself out of it. I figured if I was going to die, I didn't want to know what was happening. Well, I apparently turned into some kind of monster yelling at my older son and husband and doing really bizarre things. My mother, who is a retired Registered Nurse, finally made me go to the hospital. They did a scan and I had not caused myself any permanent deficits with the Fiorinal. I started to sober up and realize what I was doing. But the crazy thing is I kept sneaking cigarettes from people and smoking them even after I knew I must be nuts to do something like that. I was in complete denial of the situation.

By July of 1995, I pretty much had it together, and I cried every night. God, night time was the worst. In the light of day, it is easy to believe that all is okay. But at night when the house is still and you can hear every beat of your heart, the terror is unimaginable. Thank God, I could talk to my husband. I would cry and tell him how scared I was that I was going to die and that I would never see my baby grow up or feel his sweet little head on my chest. I worried about my older son even more because I didn't know how he was handling all of this and did he feel free to talk about his fears.

I went through August-November of 1995 with five more angioplasty surgeries, because they kept failing. I was seeing a doctor at that time that, in my opinion, was angioplasty happy. When in doubt angioplasty them! I started getting much smarter though and realizing that I had to take control of my own care. I dropped that doctor and started seeing a woman who was also in that practice. That is when I started feeling hope. She is very bright, young and on the forefront of women and heart disease. She tells it like it is, but with such care and concern you can't help but feel hope. Through all of this I was working as much as I could. In January of 1996, while at work, I received a call from the hospital that my 17 year old son was in a car accident. He was alive but that was all they would tell me. A friend from work drove me to the hospital where my husband met me. My son had broken his back L-3, 4,5 and his neck C-1, 2. I fell to the floor in the emergency room literally begging God to save my son. The doctor took him to surgery and he had a halo brace put on. He was then transferred to the Spinal Clinic. Believe it or not my son was out of the halo and dancing at his Prom in March of that year. God answered my prayers. But the stress of it all proved too much for me and we decided on bypass.

The doctor that was chosen to do my surgery came the night before, and hopped up on the window sill in my room and told me what he was going to do and what my chances were. I liked him immediately and when you're facing this kind of surgery, that is a big plus.

All of my brothers and sisters called to wish me well. I have five brothers and three sisters so that was a lot of talking. Plus my husband has thirteen brothers and sisters and I talked with all of them as well. I did a lot of crying that night telling my husband that if I didn't make it please let my children know how much I loved them and how sorry I was not to be there for them. The next morning, 7:00 a.m. sharp I was wheeled out for bypass.

My bypass was supposed to be a double, but one of the arteries was so full of stents that we couldn't do anything about it. I remember asking if I would have another heart attack; the doctor told me he hoped I would develop collateral blood flow first but he could not give me any guarantees. On the day I was to leave the hospital I remember watching, 90 year old men who were moving quicker than I was. Where was all this energy I was supposed to have? I went home and got progressively worse. I remember telling my husband that I would rather be dead than live like this. My husband called an ambulance for me and I was rushed back to the hospital. Lucky me I had developed Pericarditis which happens in about fifteen percent of cases. We tried treating it with Prednisone but it did no good. The symptoms I felt during angina were extremely similar to what I was now feeling. Of course my doctor was on vacation and I got stuck with the angioplasty king who sent me home. One week later, I went to the office for a routine follow up and my doctor was so upset at my appearance that she did an echo, phoned my other doctor and told him I needed an emergency Pericardial Window. She was so afraid I was going to die of cardiac tamponade before they could get it done. So one month after bypass here I am again having more surgery. It went pretty well, although I have never been able to get rid of the Pericarditis. I do not have an autoimmune problem or a connective tissue disorder or anything that would cause all of this.

My doctor finally set me up with an immunologist who I see regularly along with her. We are trying many new things and slowly making some progress on the Pericarditis. My doctor put me on medical leave permanent disability in March of 1997. Thank God for that because the stress from work wasn't helping. So now I live with what they call Dressler's Syndrome, 1 in 100,000 have it.

My yearly thallium stresses have all showed no blockages and I am grateful for whatever time I have. I think I have faced up to the fact that I have chronic illness. One thing that has gotten me through is the message board on the Internet. Especially, the message boards involving other women. For years we have been treated the same as our male counterparts. Doctors are only just now realizing that we are not the same. I see people who are much more lost and alone than I am, and it feels so good to help. My doctor and I have been discussing setting up a therapy group for her female patients.

I have two footnotes to this:

On November 7, my five-year-old, my husband and I did the walk America for the American Heart Association in Atlanta. It was really wonderful to see so many people with heart disease are out enjoying life, and all it offers.

In January of 1999, my husband, who is only 47, suffered a stroke. Thank God he is getting better and is already back at work. Apparently he has a basilar artery at the back of his neck that is abnormally small.

My oldest son is now 21, and manages a sports bar here in town. I am so proud of the man that he has become. My little boy just turned five and he is as sweet and bright a child as you could ever hope for and my wonderful husband and I just thank God that we are still here, still able to enjoy our children, family and friends and still crazy about each other.

If there is anything I want to stress in my story, it is that you are in charge of your body. If you don't feel that you are getting what you need from your doctor, fire him/her and find one that you can work with. The relationship between you and your cardiologist should be one of equality. I can't even tell you what my doctor has been to me. If I call she answers; not her nurse, not the switchboard, but her. She has great belief in my ability to know my own body so if I tell her something is wrong, then something's wrong.

Sincerely,

Mary E. Arehart

*"Then shall thy light break forth as the morning, and thine health shall spring forth speedily: and thy righteousness shall go before thee: the glory of the Lord shall be thy reward."*
*Isaiah 58:8*

*Patrick conveys his story with such truth and conviction that is serves to instill within us the importance of life as just a "whisper and a vapor" to be cherished to the fullest. Patrick, your title says it all.*

# Little Do We Know, The Frailty of Life
## By
## Patrick D. Callahan

Sunday, February 8, 1993 began as had so many before it: Sunday school and church in the morning; a relaxing afternoon and evening of reading and, probably, watching the Denver Broncos sweep to another victory; and, finally, retiring at our usual time of ten p.m. There ended the usual! Without my usual tossing and turning for an hour or so I went right to sleep only to be aroused at about midnight. I awoke with a slightly burning ache in my upper left chest. Thinking that the problem was probably heartburn I finally arose, mixed a glass of baking soda and water, and went back to bed. As might be expected, I burped a couple of times, but the ache did not go away. In fact it increased in intensity and migrated to the shoulder. At this point I ruled out heartburn and reached for the Nitroglycerin that was prescribed back in 1991, when I had experienced chest pains.

I arose, placed a tablet under my tongue and waited the prescribed fifteen minutes. No relief! Placed a couple under the tongue and waited. Still I had no relief, and the pain was coming down the left arm.

One more attempt. A couple under the tongue and again waited—no relief. At around three thirty, I decided it was time to get moving. I awoke our oldest son, who was still living with us, and asked him to take me to the Medical Center. By this time the pain had reached my left hand.

At the hospital, the emergency staff wasted no time in getting me onto a gurney, inserting IV's, beginning an EKG, and drawing blood. Results of the blood draw were quick in coming—a definite heart attack—and not the first one. I was admitted to the hospital for further evaluation and tests overnight.

Early the next morning, my doctor was at my bedside advising, me that a catherization was in order to specifically determine what needed to be done. By mid-morning, it was off to the operating room where a shunt was placed in the right groin artery. Initially the catherization wire was run up into the heart for exploratory purposes only. They found two arteries badly blocked. That determined that a balloon angio-plasty procedure needed to be preformed on each offending artery.

After a week in the hospital I was discharged, returned home, and assigned to a rehabilitation center for a specially designed program for heart patients for a period of three months. I returned to light duty work after three weeks. I was an Industrial Engineer for a machine shop so being placed on light duty presented few problems for my employer or myself; plenty of people were around to do whatever heavy lifting needed to be done. Progress seemed to be normal and I felt much better than I had in quite some time. The rehabilitation schedule called for a treadmill/thallium test the final week of the program. I failed the test! One of the arteries had again blocked. To say the least I am worried but was reassured by my doctor that the artery probably could be reopened with another angioplasty procedure.

In either late May or early June, it was back to the operating room for another angioplasty attempt. All did not go well! Somehow the artery became punctured. The procedure was called off. As is always the case with angioplasty procedures, there is a cardiac surgical team standing by should an emergency arise. My doctor and this team consulted on how to proceed. I was told that a bypass would have to be performed but that, with my consent, they would like to wait until I had regained strength. I readily agreed since we had arranged to attend a family reunion in late June. I was set up with an appointment with a surgeon for a family consultation. He was in agreement with the delay, but cautioned that should I become ill, to contact him immediately so that an operation could be scheduled.

Although I was feeling less than top drawer, we left for Missouri the third weekend of June for the family reunion. With all that takes place at these functions, I knew that once back home in Colorado I would have to make arrangements for the bypass. Back home, my doctor was contacted and he set the operation for the morning of July 10th.

Was I scared? Yes! I think I was more concerned for my family than I was for myself. They had already been through far too much and this procedure was life threatening. On the morning of July 11th, they and our pastor were by my side as I was wheeled toward the operating room. Several hours later, hooked up to a heart/lung machine, I was back in my Intensive Care room. My first recollection was that of someone slapping my face and asking me to wake up. It was one of the many "angels" that looked after my every need during both the angioplasties and the bypass. As I awoke, I wanted to breathe, but that infernal machine was there to do the job for me and wasn't about to relinquish its job. Good thing I was tied down hand and foot. Otherwise, I would have had it out of my throat! In a few hours I was allowed to breathe on my own. The medical staff knew what they were doing! As so often happens following major surgery, a spell of depression sets in. I found myself sobbing for no apparent reason. As I was trying to control my emotions, a nurse by my side told me to "let it out" that they had "beaten up on me. Looking back, that is exactly what had happened.

Another week in the hospital and it was back home to heal and recuperate. During my three hospital stays, a Mended Hearts visitor had stopped by each time to offer support and encouragement. I vowed during the last stay that when I was well enough I, too, would become involved with Mended Hearts. That day came in November of 1993. My wife, Margaret, and I have been members ever since and became Mended Hearts visitors at the local Veteran's Administration Medical Center sometime in late 1994.

Sometime in 1994, I again experienced chest pain and was taken by ambulance to the hospital (Our medical coverage had been changed to Kaiser). Procedures revealed that the bypass had grafted off. Since the mammary artery had been used to perform the bypass, and laid in such a curled position that any attempt to reopen the artery would be unsuccessful. If the artery could be reopened, approximately ten percent of the heart muscle was dead. Now, what do you do?

The answer is medication. Medication to slow the heart down. Medication to dilate the arteries. Not pleasant! It took three tries before we found prescriptions that did not leave me nauseous within an hour of taking. There is some though, that these medications and my diabetic oral medication may interact with and create some of the adverse side effects.

What precipitated all these heart problems? Looking back on my life style, I only blame myself. I was a heavy smoker—four packs a day. I ended up in a military hospital in April 1993 with lung congestion. I quit cold turkey but took a year to clear lungs of all the tars. I traded smoking for eating. I became quite overweight. In the early 80's, was diagnosed with Type II diabetes. And, to top it off, I am what some call a Type A personality—constantly on the go.

Given all that has happened and the side effects of past and present medications, I've been blessed with an additional six and one half years of useful life. I'm 67 and looking forward to several more years of productive life.

Did I get through all of this on my own? Not even close! I give great credit to a faith in my God, a very supportive family, a supportive employer, friends galore, and Mended Hearts. I was placed on a number of prayer groups from the very beginning—My doctor is a firm believer, that those with a strong faith survive and recover from these procedures far better than those who have doubts. Margaret and our three terrific children have been my staunch supporters and those who have pulled me up short when I, obviously, was trying to do too much or going at a pace too great.

I've been retired now for the past three and one half years. No, I haven't taken to my easy chair full time! There is far too much to be done. In addition to volunteer work with Mended Hearts, The American Legion, Masonic Lodge, membership in a garden club and stamp club, we manage to travel some each year. In June 1998 we spent the month in England, the home of my wife. July-August 1999 found us on the road to Vancouver, British, Columbia, and on board the Rhapsody of the Seas cruise liner for a seven day inside cruise along the coast of British Columbia and Alaska. Homeward via Olympic Peninsula for a visit with our youngest son, and then home across Washington, Oregon, Utah and Colorado. Add a couple of family reunions to that, and you have better than 10,000 miles of driving. No, we are not sitting still. What few remaining years we have left, we plan to enjoy family and friends.

What are we, my wife and I, seeing as we visit with heart patients at the Veterans' Medical Center? Mainly men ranging in age from their late 30s to well over 80. Most undergo bypass procedure and are back home or transferred to a support facility within a week. Those who have a support group, family, and/or friends at home recover the quickest. There are those who have no one at home to care for them and must go to nursing facility of some sort. The latter are the ones who recover the slowest and have the deepest depression. Sometimes we can get them needed help through the hospital's Social Services section. Then there are those with life style issues: diabetes, obesity, and smokers. Aside from the diabetes, for which they are already being treated, Mended Hearts through the American Heart Association provides counseling and materials on dieting, exercise and the impact of smoking on both lung and heart disease. Where possible, we visit with the family of the patient in an effort to prepare them for the in-hospital care and what to expect once their loved one returns home. The motto of Mended Hearts, Inc. is, "It's Great to be Alive—and to Help Others." So be it!

*"Bless the Lord, O my soul: and all that is within me, bless his holy name."*
*"Bless the Lord, O my soul, and forget not all his benefits:*
*Who forgiveth all thine iniquities; who healeth all thy diseases;*
*Who redeemeth thy life from destruction; who crowneth thee with loving kindness and tender mercies."*
*Psalm 103: 1-4*

# Beverly Brinkman's Experience

25 November 1999

I had a heart attack on December 4, 1996, the same day that I retired from the railroad after 41 years. I had been having a strange radiating ache for four or five days. It started between my shoulder blades went up to my shoulders and down the top of both arms to my fingers. It would come and go but for some reason on Monday afternoon I decided I'd better get it checked out. I really thought it was gall bladder or hiatus hernia. I got an appointment for 5 p.m. with a doctor I'd never seen. In fact, I hadn't been to a doctor for twenty years. Why should I ever think "heart attack?" I was female, 62 years old, post menopausal, overweight, under exercised (in fact, no exercise is a better way to put it), and I smoked. I had been smoking for 42 years. I had my last cigarette in the doctor's office parking lot before I went in. He asked me some questions, took my blood pressure, listened to my heart, and called a nurse in to give me an EKG. He came back in two minutes, said "lie down, put this under your tongue (Nitro), you're having a heart attack." I laughed and started to sit up and he pushed me back down. He said, "I've called 911 and they should be here shortly. They kept giving me more Nitro until we got to the hospital because that ache wouldn't go away. The cardiologist at the hospital decided against the clot busters because they weren't sure when the attack had started. I whined and whined, "This is my retirement day. I'm supposed to go out for dinner." They ended up giving me morphine because the pain still didn't completely go—away but I think it was to shut me up. The next morning, they transferred me to another hospital for an angiogram. It showed that I had one completely blocked artery on the back of my heart that already had collateral blood vessels, and that the heart tissue was dead so no balloon and no surgery. They would treat me with medicine. I was in the hospital for a week and had a thallium stress test the last day to make sure the heart muscle was dead. It was. Both doctors told me that if I wanted to die in 18 months or less, to just keep smoking. When I got home, the first thing I did was take a shower and wash my hair. I couldn't take one in the hospital because of the cardiac monitor attached to me. I thought I might die from dirty hair but the doctor said, "No" The woman I live with does not smoke and she had cleared out all cigarettes, lighters, ashtrays, etc. I knew that I could never take even one puff of a cigarette for the rest of my life. For the first month I wasn't around anyone that smoked, so that made it easier. So far in almost three years, I'm still hanging in there. I don't even think about it any more, but know it's still a danger to me.

When I left the hospital, I had three prescriptions to get filled, plus a baby aspirin. My blood pressure was very hard to control. At each doctor visit he added another pill. I'm now on Sular, Metoprolol, Covera HS, Prinivil, Lasix, Levoxyl, and Zocor. I feel pretty good now but get tired easily and have short-term memory loss. I blame Metoprolol for both of these side effects but I guess they aren't too bad.

The best thing that happened to me was Cardiac Rehab. I was horrified at first, and scared that I wouldn't be able to do anything, but the nurses were so nice. I learned so much about diet and life style changes, and three years later, I still go once a month. I used to think that reading a heavy book was exercise but now I have my own treadmill and I think I'm addicted to it. I don't feel right going out if I don't exercise first.

Diet has been harder, but I've managed to lose 30 pounds. I need to lose another 30 but it comes off so slowly. I switched to as much low fat or no fat food that I could, and it's amazing how many good things there are out there. For the first year after my attack, I was afraid to go more than 50 miles away from my doctor but we go all over now. I have an active, normal life and I'm probably in a lot better shape than I would have been without the heart attack.

Beverly

*Carson took all the pre-exercise precautions, which most likely turned out to be a blessing for him. He relates his coronary artery bypass experience to show that many symptoms of heart disease are atypical even in men.*

# Carson Klitz

So here goes. I am now nearly 62, and a white male weighing 207. At age 55, I weighed 240 and decided to start to run. I had a stress test and was approved to run, which I did. Never ran fast, but ran 20 miles per week. I ran the week prior to May 16, and had a burning sensation in my chest, which I attributed to paint remover I had been using in restoring a Model T Ford. On May 16 1999, while running, I had burning in my chest. I had to walk to the car. That evening around 2000 hrs, I got severe pain in my chest that ran to left arm (but not down the arm). Pain passed in a minute or two, so I assumed I was cured. It was not so. In ten minutes or so, pain returned as before. This time I drove myself to our small rural hospital and complained of chest pain. My local doctor gave me Nitro and called Springfield (they do hundreds of heart operations a year) and the cardiologist on duty advised me to take two aspirins and see him in the morning. My doctor called the other hospital, and the cardiologist said send him over—pdq. That is just what they did.

The next morning, I had five bypasses. Blockage was from seventy-five percent to ninety nine percent. Everything went okay, but two days post op, I had atrial flutter. It converted with medication. All went well, and I went home that Friday.

On June 24, my surgeon gave me a complete release to do anything. That afternoon while working, I had atrial flutter again, and it was back to the hospital where it was converted shortly. I had no problems until

June 29, when I woke up at 0500, and you guessed it, atrial flutter. It converted itself (my cardio said it probably would) and since that time I have been trouble free.

Prior to my MI, my heart rate was around 60 while resting and now with metoprolol it is in the high 40's. I went to rehab and still do. Also stress tests permitted me to run again, which I do on my off days from rehab. I feel better that I have for years and I do anything from cutting hedge posts to driving a tractor for 12 hours.

For many years, I have suffered from PVC's and I still do. I am more fearful than before with them, but I guess I am doing really well.

I hope that I never have to repeat the operation, but if I have not other choice, I would do it in a minute. I hope this has been of some help.

Carson Klitz

*Heart Disease experiences are as different as people. Sparky shares his story in a way that is both very serious and at the same time, uplifting and entertaining. His writing is a pleasure to read though his disease is not.*

*"Greater is he that is in you, than he that is in the world."*
*1 John 4:4*

# Heart Disease Ain't Easy—Sparky

Several years ago, I retired from the U.S. Air Force. I had been noticing a tired, lethargic feeling for some time. With diagnosed hypertension, I thought that was the problem. Many medications later, the high B/P was still not in good control. The angina was getting worse and the military doctors were trying to find the cause. Treadmill, Thallium stress test, echocardiogram, and many EKGs later—all were normal. They could not find a cause or problem. Why could they not find out what was wrong? Put me on Prilosec for heartburn. This didn't help at all. Throughout the next two to three years, the pain increased in the chest. The doctor finally gave me nitroglycerin just as a precaution!

Oh, how I wondered what was going on? My dad died at 49 with a tumor and mom at 53 with a second heart attack. All that is going through my mind is that I won't live to see 49 years old. In 1999, I'm now 45. I thought of all the bad things I've done. I smoked 3 packs a day for many years but quit that in 1986. I thought I'd done well for myself, but little did I know the consequences. During the winter of 1998 and summer of 1999, the pains kept getting worse. Doctors just keep saying to not worry about it.

Pains were getting severe in the summer of 1999. I was actually afraid to take the nitroglycerin. I had heard that it would give you a really bad headache. And if I took the Nitro, that was a sign that I needed help or hospitalization, right? I never did take any Nitro, still haven't till this day. I didn't even take it when I lay in bed one morning with chest pains that made me sick. Blood pressure of 182/122 and pain in both arms. But let me lay here a little while, I'll be okay. Okay, I've got an idea! If I take double my blood pressure medication that should bring the blood pressure down! Okay, take the pills. I can feel it working, an hour later I feel much better. Even good enough to go to work! That's it, just take twice the number of pills and I'll feel fine. I thought a few days later that maybe I should tell the doctor. I had an appointment to see the mental health doctor. I'd seen him a few times for depression. I don't really think he figured me out.

That day, I went over to see my internal medicine doctor. "Oh shoot, he's on vacation." They suggest I go to the emergency room if I'm having chest pains. But I'm not having any pain, I feel fine. Maybe that's because I'd been doubling my BP medicines. My wife firmly suggested we should go over to the emergency room, so I followed her lead. The emergency room people went spastic! I kept telling them I felt fine right then. They finally got me back into the emergency room and started in on me. First was ECG: abnormal—showed inverted T wave. So next were the blood tests. I felt so sorry for the poor little nurse that put the IV in my hand. Panic attacks with needles are my specialty. I about liked to thrown her across the emergency room! Through much frustration and patience, she finally gets it in. She draws about 14 gallons of blood and starts the testing. The emergency room was extremely busy that day and the testing took forever.

The next thing I knew, there was a Major standing in front of me (yes, a military hospital). He says he's got some good news and bad news. Good news is that I'm alive and in the hospital, bad news is that I've had a heart attack in the last few days. He wants to admit me and run some tests. Okay, here we go! Up to Intensive Care Unit, and hooked me up to every machine available! I really can't figure it out. I feel fine, and all these other people are in really bad shape. They do test after test.

The next day they come to get me for a heart catherization. I'd heard of these and knew it involved needles—Oh boy! I was sent down to the catherization lab, with wife beside me all the way. When she kissed me and said she'd see me in a little while, that is the first time I felt fear pulse through me. Show the fear—never! Into the lab and the doctor was explaining it. All I wanted was to be unconscious. Then came the shot in addition to the IV. I faintly remember a few things they asked me to do but basically nothing. The next thing I remember is being in the hallway with my wife. I lay on the table, waiting on the doctor. He came out and again, some good news, and some bad news. Bad news is that I've had two heart attacks. I have one hundred percent blockage on right and left coronary arteries, and ninety percent and sixty percent on two others. Good news is they can bypass these. I'm thinking to myself, a bypass, open-heart surgery is good news? They wheel me back to intensive care. I remember being fairly quiet on the way. My wife was fighting back tears, which kind of made me want to cry. Many things going through my mind, especially my mother and especially my father, who died at 49.

Later that day they told me that they would transfer me to a hospital downtown for the bypass. With the military cutbacks, they didn't have heart surgeons anymore. So later that day, I was transferred to a step down room to wait three days for Monday to go downtown. The weekend took forever. They did let me walk around a little with my telemetry unit on. What a long, long weekend I experienced?

Okay Monday is here, time to take the ride downtown. Wow, they load me up in an ambulance and everything. What a rough ride in the in the ambulance? We get to the other hospital and the paperwork starts. I get a room with an older bypass patient. He's waiting for his son to come and get him. I really just want to be alone now. I'm starting to think about everything—doesn't help. I get visits from EVERYBODY! My wife, kids, preacher, nurses, doctors, co-workers, hey it's a parade!

The doctor comes in and explains the procedure, he does seem very confident in himself. He has done thousands of bypasses, wow! Later that night, the nurses come in with the electric razors. Oh, how I hate this. I'm such a hairy person. There go the legs, arms, and the very hairy chest. Oh no, they even got to change the blades it's so bad! And don't you know that right in the middle of all this, in comes a female co-worker—oh how embarrassing!

The surgery is first thing in the morning. Everyone leaves and now I am alone. I'm so worried, but will only let it show to myself. Be strong, especially for my wife. I cry that night again thinking of my dad and what would happen to my wife if anything happens. The sleep that night is extremely restless. About 5:30 a.m., the nurse comes in for me to take my morning shower. I go down the hallway to the shower room. I feel so lonely again. The room is so cold, barren, and lifeless. After the short shower, back to the room where they start preparing me. All I want is to be unconscious now. I'm scared to death, but let it show— never! My wife shows up with the kids and her sister. I now feel better with family surrounding me. I feel like I'm in a daze. Trying to block out anything happening. I kissed my wife and hugged everyone on the way to surgery. Memories blur from there.

The next memory I have is waking up in recovery, CCU. On no! I can't breathe! I have something down my throat. I go into a panic attack! I can't breathe! I can't breathe! I thrash about violently. The nurse kept telling me to settle down, settle down. I can't reach the tube with my hands. I don't understand why I can't reach this thing in my throat? Later I realize my arms are tied down to the sides of the bed. As the nurse starts to leave, I feel as though I'm dying! Tears roll down my checks; I am afraid, and panicking. I start kicking the bed as hard as I can with my feet. Knock the bed apart! Then they'll listen to me. The nurse came back and again told me to settle down. I think, "doesn't she know I'm dying?" I kick harder and harder. Get this out of my throat NOW! More kicking, and more kicking. They finally come in and removed the tube. Ahhhh! I can breathe but they are worried as my respiration slows. Maybe that tube shouldn't have come out.

The next thing I know, they let my wife back to see me. My first words to her were, "This sucks," and "I feel like I've been run over by a herd of Mack Trucks." I could see the concern and horror in my wife's eyes. I know I looked a site with tubes running out of me everywhere and swollen up like a giant panda bear. I know my wife wanted to cry but she held back the tears for me. Then I had my wife and daughter at my side. They said I liked to have squeezed their hands off. I really didn't know I was doing that.

Then some of the pain medication started to wear off. I was becoming more coherent but very uncomfortable. I was turning into a real grouch! I asked my wife to fluff my pillow. She said maybe they wanted me to lay a certain way and she shouldn't do that. Boy, did I get mad. Just fluff the d… thing! I know I didn't feel very good. They said to not be afraid to ask for pain medication and I wasn't. But what they were giving me wasn't making the pain go away. I asked the nurse for more and finally she gave me something that really put me in la-la land. My wife, daughter, and sister-in-law were still around as I was in and out of sleeping. The rest of the day was a struggle just to stay comfortable. It seems like time just stood still. I would doze awhile and wake and ask what time it was—10 minutes later. Lots of medicines and lots of blood work. Thank goodness for the IV they took the blood out of. No more needles in me! Then came the first night, the first long, long night! Every hour, wake me up, take blood pressure, take this pill, draw blood, and check on me. What a long, long night it is? At 6 a.m., the nurse came in and did BP checks. She cheerily said that the next hour they'd be in to get me up. I thought I was dreaming and dozed back off.

At 7 a.m., the nurse came in the room and announced, "It's time to get up!" Okay, I thought she meant wake up so I did. "Get up," she repeated. But nurse, "I don't think you understand I just had open-heart surgery yesterday." I said. "We know, remember that we're your nurses, now it's time to get up out of bed," she said. Fear ran throughout my body. I can't get up; I'm in too much pain! "Okay, let's teach you how to get up out of bed." she said. Oh no, I thought. They're going to hurt me. "Now, just roll over like this, position your bed, and use this arm to slightly aid in pushing up." she explained. Wow, it was a breeze, and they were right. Slow, now, very slow, I make it over to the chair and sit down. I'm actually sitting in a chair at 7 a.m. the next morning after open-heart surgery. You've got to be kidding, I think. I sit in the chair over an hour. I watched some TV and start using my breathing machine. I can hardly get the thing to work. I'm still very weak and tired. But sitting in the chair surprisingly makes me feel better. After 8 a.m., I work my way back to bed and tenderly get in, slowly wiggling my way back to comfort and doze off.

Oh here they come again, time to eat. I never had a problem with eating. I would eat everything they gave me, as I had a big appetite. I've heard of many others who could not eat, but me. Then came more prodding, poking, blood work, you name it. I still was experiencing much pain, so I kept asking for the pain medications, they helped a lot. The constant barrage of doctors, nurses, and staff just kept coming. Finally, they told me I was headed for a step down room. It is much better now—It's is just like a regular room.

The breathing and coughing exercises are very important. So is getting up and sitting up and moving. The more I did the more they helped. Started feeling better immediately. Sure the pain was still there. It hurt badly, but nothing I could handle. It was still very hard for me to imagine what had happened to me. I mean, they had stopped my heart for over 2 hours to do the quadruple bypass. That amazed me. The thought of dying was fading from me fast, I knew I was actually going to live!

The remainder of the day was routine. As nighttime got there, they brought a roll-a-way bed in for my wife. That made me feel so secure knowing she was there with me. I was safe and sound with her. Until they started in again, every two hours. Blood pressure checks, medicine, etc. Wake up, it's time for something anything. I couldn't get any rest. Then at 4 a.m. a male nurse came in. "Wake up." he said, "Huh, what?" I thought "Wake up, it's time to weigh you." "WHAT! You've got to be kidding me? Get out of my room! You don't wake a person at 4 a.m. to weigh them!" "Oh yea we do." "Please get up so I can weigh you." he stated. Begrudgingly, I get up and get on the scales. I go back to bed and instantly to sleep.

The second day is better. I feel much better and even get to go for walk with the rehab people. That afternoon, I attend rehab with another guy. These are simple exercises while you're sitting in a chair. A little walk, and its back to the room. I get up and walk a lot this day. The wife is a tremendous help—Loads of encouragement! Until she tried to hurt me. Yea, I'd been up sitting in the chair eating. I still had two chest tubes and a catheter, in with all the boxes, bags, and equipment to go along with it. While in the chair, we hung the bag from the catheter on the back of the chair. Once done eating, I made my way back to the bed. I rolled the machine for the chest tubes back bedside and she scooted the chair back across. "NO WAIT, I'm hooked up to that bag on the chair in a very precarious way!" I screamed. She just about jerked me and my lifeline out of the bed. "Oh I'm sorry, I'm sorry, I'm sorry!" she apologized. It was the awaking of my life! Okay, everything is still installed. I'm okay! Whew, what a scare. We joke about this a lot now.

Day 3—The doctor says I might be able to go home today. I'm really afraid to go though. Here I have all the protection of the nurses (except they didn't protect me from my wife yesterday) and if anything should happen I'm at the hospital, not 80 miles away. Oh well, I'm getting discharged, but it's hurry up and wait. I've got to do this test, talk to this person, etc. Finally, I'm wheeled out to the car. My wife carefully loaded my tons of flowers and me in the car. She drives, oh so carefully home. I'm hugging the heck out of my heart pillow to keep my chest from hurting. Finally, home and exhausted. I sat on the couch and then reclined some, just like the hospital bed. I can't get comfortable. I try to sleep that night on the recliner part of couch. I bet I get a whole two to three hours of sleep.

The next day, I move my recuperating head quarter's upstairs. I move, Oh so slow! But now I'm in a better recliner. I have everything I need TV, bathroom, etc. I sleep much better in this recliner and everything is very convenient. Now the slow job of recuperation starts. I must remember to do my aerobic and breathing exercises. The breathing exercises are like a game—how high can I make the little ball go? At least this way I am doing it many more times a day than I'm supposed to. I'm tired, so very, very tired. I tend to drift off to sleep at the drop of a hat. But I realize this is good for me and it's what I'm supposed to be doing.

Days pass good ones and bad ones. I start coughing a little more. The pain! I hold my heart pillow tight against the chest, as it seems everything is coming apart every time I cough. My heart pillow reminds me of Linus' security blanket he carries around in the Charlie Brown Peanuts cartoon. I carry my pillow everywhere, just afraid what might happen if I didn't have it. I even sleep with it held tight to my chest! I can remember the first time I rode in the car. We passed over a railroad track that angled across the road. The tracks were pretty rough and at a slow speed tossed the car from side to side. I was taken by surprise and it felt like by ribs were rubbing up and down on each other. Of course, I screamed in pain and my wife thought she had killed me. She apologized and apologized but it was just another lesson learned. There are many lessons.

My first walking experience came on a bright, sunny, beautiful day. Being the big strong man, I figure I've got this licked. I'm going to walk down to the lake and back (about 400 yards one way). I get my pepper spray for dogs, in case I have a problem, and the wife and I head on out. Moving pretty, slow, no, real slow, as we make our way along. I can do this; I've been home now a whole week! Moving slower now, I'm starting to get winded, slower now. Maybe we should turn around, yep, turn around. But I've only gone 75 yards! Who cares, turn around! We start back and I've never realized that the road slants uphill slightly to my house. Slightly heck! Although it's only about 2 or 3-degree incline, but it looked like the Rocky Mountains to me. Moving even slower now, I start thinking about having the wife go get the car. No, I can't ask her that, I keep walking. Finally, we make it back to the house. I sit down exhausted. Get a drink and take a nap. Don't worry it'll get better.

I slowly learn to do things again, and learn what things not to do. Sure honey, I'll help you wax the car. After all, it's been 3 weeks since the surgery and I'm bored. It won't hurt me to help since we just got one of those new electric buffers. Buff, buff, and buff, away. After an hour or so, we are done. Inside again, I sit down feeling pretty good that I had done something. Later that evening, the stiffness and pain sit in. Oh why was I stupid enough to do something like that? I pay for it by being sore for the next three days.

It's now three months later. I'm in Cardiac Rehab Phase 2 at my local hospital. My nurses are the greatest. They have taken care of me and helped nurture me both mentally and physically back to health again. Cardiac Rehab is one of the most important things anyone can do for their self. You do preventative maintenance on your car don't you? That's all it is, preventative maintenance for your heart, mind, and body.

Talking about your mind, Oh my, let's talk about something I feel is very important—mind support. You WILL get depressed, and at some time or another depression will affect you. You are not alone, believe me. You have to have somebody to talk to. I felt like nobody in the world understood how I felt, and that depressed me more. The best thing I ever did was log into a website called WebMD. It has message boards and chat rooms for heart patients. I could actually have conversations with other people like me. I learned that what I was going through was actually normal. And by me lending an ear and support to other scared heart patients, that actually helped me tremendously.

Lastly, we shall talk about one thing that will help a person more than anything. It's called, "ATTITUDE." Can you remember the saying, "With God, all things are possible." "It's true, it's attitude." Ever see an ant push something 10 times his size? It's attitude. How about David and Goliath? It's attitude. And how about that drop of rain, that after that much work, carved the Grand Canyon. If a raindrop could have it, it's attitude. A person controls their actions and attitudes as they wish. I've seen some people, and we've all done it, who want others to feel sorry for them. Bologna! Get off your tuff and help yourself! But at least have the support group that will back you up. When you do get depressed, talk to somebody. Just don't sit around and cry about it.

Okay, so you've got heart disease. So do one heck of a lot of the rest of us. And to tell the truth, I don't care! I'm going to take care of myself so I can enjoy my grandkids, children, wife, and life!

Good Luck and God Bless!

Sparky

*Heart disease strikes the young. Sandy is a young woman who is vivacious, loving and fights her illness on a daily basis. She exhibits the inner strength and courage to help other heart patients' "demand" the best medical care available.*

# Sandy Martin

14 November 1999

It was a Saturday and I was eating dinner when the pain began. First, a sharp one, a gripping chest pain, like, someone squeezed the life out of me. I told my husband that something was wrong. Laughing he said, "Why are you having a heart attack?" Then I saw his ashen face as I said, "it's possible." He rushed me to the local emergency room and the triage nurse poo—pooed me with her disapproving looks.

My blood pressure was not high and I was not diaphoretic. "Well," I stated." "I am a nurse and I say something is wrong." "A little gas," she says to my husband, as I stated "gas does not affect my left arm, I want a doctor and I am not leaving until you do a EKG." She was less than thrilled with me and so was my husband. I guess I was a bit embarrassing. Well the doc came and spoke with me, and started to run an EKG and enzymes. Sure enough there, it is the beginning of my nightmare. The test showed major blockages occurring. The doctor approached me like Marcus Welby, holding my hands and telling me that I had some severe problems. The tears ran down my face, "I am a nurse," I heard myself say. "How could I not have known?" I had one at ninety five percent, ninety percent, eighty five percent and seventy five percent blockages. They were transporting me to a hospital that did bypasses. I am in the ambulance asking my nurse if I would make it. Scared was not the word for it. This was the longest journey of my life. Next morning, I was going through a triple bypass. I was awakening in

ICU and I could not talk; I wanted water. The nurse was telling my husband not much ice, she may want it, but she will vomit. I begged for ice or water. A tube was in my throat and I felt tubes everywhere. I lay there and thought, "I did die." I heard everyone and watched while my surgery was performed. I really did, but I never told anyone, they would not believe me I am sure. A few days later, the chest tubes came out. Well, when a doctor tells you something will not hurt rest assured it will. I delivered a child through my chest, to say the least.

Then they tell me I am good for 20 years. I was in the hospital for 10 long days. Coming home was just the beginning of all my problems. My incision dehisced, got infected and guess what? Twenty-one days later I am having chest pains again. While I was home I cried a lot, got depressed, and watched myself in the mirror waiting for my carotid artery to stop beating. It looked like it was gonna pulse out of my body any minute. Self-esteem was none. My breasts were crooked now with its stitching. I was scared from my clavicle to below my breasts, I have quite a few drainage holes, and I thought, "Who will want me?" Sexy was now just a word. My husband tried to assure me, but the nicer he was the more I thought it was pity. Then the arteries collapsed and 4 stents were put in. Well, the stents restenosed, a few times, and they figured out something else was wrong here. My cardiologist sent me to Washington D.C. where they were doing some new experiments on re-stenoses with stents. I had brachytherapy radiation to the stents. So many times I restenosed. Chest pain is a normal now. I prayed this worked. So far it has. I am still having chest pains, but no blockages for now. I have reached a new plateau in life.

I was not to expect anything. Every day above ground is a plus. With all the drugs

I am on, I do not know which way is up anymore—but they keep me alive. We are looking at the blood now; think it is a coagulation factor causing all my problems.

I say "yeah right." The only time I feel good is when I talk to other heart patients or I go to the hospital and tell heart patients what they are really in for. No one told me about all the emotional turmoil. It hurts worse than the physical pain. I feel old, unattractive, scarred and wonder each day if today will kill me. I get through the day with the sense I have helped someone get through this. So when people say I am crazy or depressing, I sure agree, but it keeps me fighting for life. I am now changing nursing fields from geriatrics to cardiac. They need me— someone needs me—thats what I live for. Everyday is a struggle because I never am pain free for a day. I pray we get to the bottom of it, but I am my own best medicine, I am the caregiver, I am the soul of nursing, I a.m. a fighter and that keeps me alive. If you ever want a friend to turn his back just tell them how you really feel. They will say "You will get through it, you are strong." Well maybe I am not! Come back! Talk to me," "Listen" "gotta run." This is what friends do. My friends are on line, they listen, we share, we care and they are always there.

Sandy Martin

> *"For he shall give his angels charge over thee, to keep thee in all thy ways."*
> *Psalms 91:11*

# Toni Emery

14 Nov 1999

I began having chest pains in June of 1997; I went to a little small town doctor who said it was just stress and gave he me some tranquilizers. I went back three more times, and he still said it was stress (Of course me being a woman and 49 it couldn't be anything else). I finally went to my regular doctor because the chest pains had gotten more frequent and I was afraid. My doctor had run an EKG and yelled at me that I should have come sooner, and that he was picking up something on the EKG. So off to a cardiologist, who ran a thallium stress test on me of which I failed to even make it two minutes. He in turn sent me to a bigger town to the hospital, where an angiogram revealed I needed a triple bypass immediately. I, of course, was horrified, scared and a mass of tears. This was all happening to fast. Wait a minute! I have a life, responsibilities! We had started my dream of having my own cafe the fall before and I had employees and much to do. Oh please God, what is this? My husband and family were beside themselves. And I still didn't understand how very serious this was, especially the fact that it involved my left main, left circumflex and right interior. The Red Cross sent for my son in the Army and off I went to surgery.

The terror I woke up to being hooked to a ventilator. Each time my husband or son came into the Intensive Care Unit the ventilator would go crazy. Get this out of me, my mind screamed. But soon it was removed and I was on my way to recovery in the hospital. Then my son went back to the Army and I was soon riding down the road towards home. But I just couldn't feel better.

First, I had a little infection in my sternum. Then, when I went for my 6 weeks check up, the cardiologist did a stress test and found out that two of the bypasses had failed. My world came crashing down around me. I would go in again and they would try to redo the bypass. Instead they cut into the left ventricle of my heart and had to close me up again. The horror of not being fixed and a doctor not sitting down and explaining to "me" what was going on in plain English, to me is a crime. I heard everything second hand, through my family. And only what they thought I needed to hear at the time. Part of the time I could tell that they weren't telling me the whole story. And to this day I know that was a real mistake. I want the truth. The surgeon said that he couldn't do anymore for me. But I didn't understand that. And my husband was in denial. But bless his heart, when they tried to release me to go home to die, he wouldn't let them. So with a fight I got angioplasty and here I am today.

I have serious Coronary Artery Disease and have had four angioplasties and my left carotid done, but I thank God each day that I am alive! I lost my café, but I got to live so my life goes on in different directions. And still when I get some angina, the fear comes rolling back. I am terrified of going to the hospital and have to take drugs at night to keep the "scaries" away. I never am able to forget that some day I'll have to go back again, but do the best I can to have a peaceful and happy life finding new directions all the time. I am letting my spirit soar for the first time, and smelling the air and the roses.

Toni Emery

*The diagnosis of Heart Disease, as told by Angela in her own words, enlightens us to the fact that life can abruptly come to a halt, as we know it. Fear is the common denominator that makes us all vulnerable to denial. God truly watches over his children in times of need, protecting us from ourselves. You can live a rewarding life after the diagnosis of heart disease. Angela proves this on a daily basis with her inspiration for others.*

# My Story
## By
## Angela Festa

My story began in February of 1998 when I was forced to visit the doctor because of an apparent bout with bronchitis. I was feeling very congested combined with periods of heart palpitations which were increasing in frequency. When these palpitations occurred, it felt like my heart would come to a sudden stop and it filled me with a sense of dread. The doctor treated me for the bronchitis using antibiotics and cough medicine. He said that the palpitations were most likely caused by the congestion, but if it continued after I had completed the medicine; I was to come back.

The medicine seemed to help a little, but after a while the palpitations returned. This time, they were worse and occurred more frequently than before. I returned to the doctor and he ordered a 24-hour holter monitor test to help determine what the problem might be. The results came back and he informed me there had been over 700 episodes of erratic heartbeats in that 24-hour period. He advised me to see a cardiologist. I was never expecting anything to be wrong with my heart. There couldn't be anything wrong with my heart. After all, I was only 36 years old! I was very afraid of going to the cardiologist. I am the mother of two teenage boys who need to have a mother very much.

When I went to see the cardiologist, he performed a treadmill stress test to determine if the palpitations are related to my heart. I lasted less than four minutes because of the chest pain. I tried to explain that the chest pain was due to my asthma, and this is common when I exerted myself. He wasn't so sure that it was asthma, and he recommended that I have additional tests. A treadmill stress test is just an overall measurement of how well the body is working. He recommended that I have either a nuclear stress test, which would show the parts of the heart having a problem, or a catheter, which would show any blockages in my arteries. The catheter was minor surgery, and the nuclear stress test was not. The nuclear stress test could show that the heart was not functioning well, but still not identify why, and I would wind up having the catheter anyway.

On May 29, 1998 I decided to have the catheter performed. Following the procedure, the doctor came in and informed me I had heart disease. I had a total of seven blocked arteries ranging from fifty percent to ninety percent blocked. He said I needed to have surgery because I was very ill. That day in May, my world came crumbling down. I did not even begin to understand what was to come, because I was in such denial of the whole situation. The very next day I quit smoking cigarettes—after 20 years of smoking a pack a day or more. I have not had a cigarette since May 30,1998, which has been very hard since my husband still smokes.

At my next appointment with the cardiologist I was informed that I needed a quadruple bypass. I immediately responded that I wanted a second opinion. He understood because he could see how depressed I was and in such a state of denial. In the meantime, he started me on several medications and recommended I begin a cardiac rehab exercise program.

When I started the rehab program, I felt very self-conscious because I was the youngest one there. I was embarrassed because it felt as though everyone was staring, and wondering, what was wrong with me. I never felt so alone as when I exercised in that rehab class. All of the "older people" were exercising at a faster rate and progressing quicker than I was. I would stick with the heart rate they put me at no matter how much pain I was in. Believe me, I was in so much pain, but I always blamed it on the Asthma. I would go home and cry because I had such a hard time keeping up with the program they put me on.

My husband and I would go for walks at night and I would always have to take little stops because of the chest pain. Of course, this was the asthma acting up. It couldn't be my heart—after all, I was too young for heart disease.

Over the next several months, I saw three more cardiologists never believing what the one before had said. Of course they all said the same thing: "SURGERY". I was in such pain and so miserable because I could no longer do simple things that I once did. I finally decided I really needed to have the operation. I could no longer deny it. The choice was to have the operation or die; so I chose to live. Not only for myself, but also for my family, because I lived in a house full of men that really needed a woman, a mother, and a wife.

Telling my mother and siblings was very hard. They could not believe what was happening to me. Not only were they upset for me, but they were also very scared wondering if this was going to happen to them next. I had no idea that there was a family history of heart disease. My mother gave me a list of family members that had heart ailments, and none of them are living. This fact was not all that comforting to me.

It was mid-October before I finally decided that I was going to have the bypass surgery. I did not want to know any details of what was about to happen to me. Someone at rehab slipped and started to talk about how they crack your chest open, and that's when it was all over for me. I broke down and started to cry uncontrollably in the middle of the exercise room. I had no idea that they actually did that. I was scared beyond belief. I think that is when it really hit me on how serious this was and I began to wonder would if I would really survive this operation. My nerves were totally shattered—I became an emotional wreck. It was very hard to function and maintain a positive attitude with the pending surgery. I think the one thing that did help was that I continued exercising from June through October, so I was in better shape than when I first found out about the heart disease. Since, I was fit, it was to my advantage, plus, I have not had a cardiac event, which could have damaged to my heart muscle.

Well there I was, the big day before the surgery. Thinking back on it, that was probably the worst day of my life. You're not sure if this will be the last day you spend with your family, and of course, they're not sure if this is their last day with you either. We spent a wonderful day doing all the things I like, which included eating my favorite meal of Kentucky Fried Chicken. There was so much love on that day that I knew I would make it. I had to make it because my family needed me.

The Medical Center was kind enough to put us up in a motel the night before surgery because we lived three hours from the hospital. So, in the morning we only had to go five minutes down the road. During that brief drive, I was very scared but calm at the same time. I was going to be healthy again, something that I have missed for a very long time now.

When we got to the hospital, they took me right into a preparation room and immediately gave me drugs. I don't even remember leaving that room. The next thing I knew, I was waking up and the surgery was over. It wound up that they only felt I needed a triple bypass. They took veins from my legs and a mammary artery from my chest. The relief that it was finally over was so great. The look in my family's eyes was overwhelming. I was alive! I had made it!

Following the surgery, I was very upset at what they had done to my body. I never really expected the incisions to be so ugly. I felt so ugly. How was my husband ever going to love me or even make love to me looking like this? I called myself the "Bride of Frankenstein." The scars were something that had never even occurred to me. You are not only scarred physically, but you are also scarred emotionally. They say when you have heart disease you are not suppose to have stress. How in the world can you not get stressed?

Recovery was not as bad as I had thought it would be. Of course they give you plenty of morphine, which helps for the pain. I was out of bed and walking around the Cardiac Unit the day after surgery. There was a little bit of drainage coming from the incision in my chest but that was all. The doctors wanted me to go home on the third day following the surgery, but I told them I would feel more comfortable if I could stay one more day.

The day after I got home we went shopping. Yes, shopping! I have to remind you that this is only six days after having a triple bypass. I had to walk slowly, but at least I was out and about. The incision on my chest was still seeping, a little more than before.

On the sixth day, I became very ill and almost collapsed. I told my husband that I needed to go to the hospital because something was very wrong. I was in the Chest Pain Emergency Unit for more than four hours when the cardiologist on duty said there was nothing wrong with my heart and I was to go see my doctor the as soon as possible. When I saw my cardiologist the next morning, he knew something was wrong. He looked at my chest and called the medical center and told them I was coming back up there. He did not let on how bad I really was.

Three hours later, I was back at the medical center; the last place in the world that I want to be. I was admitted at the emergency room and a surgical team was called down to look at me. Then they called the surgeon who had performed my bypass. I could not believe what they were about to do. They took a scalpel and cut my chest open, without warning, let alone any painkillers or anesthesia. My chest was filled with infection that came seeping out. I found out that I had a staph infection, and they were not sure how far it had traveled. It may have gone into my sternum.

I was admitted back into the hospital, where I was to stay for nine of the most miserable days in my life. I started on antibiotics and my chest wound was left open for 7 days. Three teams of doctors and three different nurses on the various shifts packed and unpacked the gauze in my chest to keep the infection drained. Talk about being depressed; I couldn't even describe the way I felt. I kept thinking, "Why could this be happening to me?" Didn't I already go through enough? What did I do so wrong in my life to deserve this? How could God make me go through this? I had so many questions and very few answers. On the eighth day, I underwent surgery again to make sure the infection was completely out. The infection had not traveled very deep, so I was spared any bone or tissue reconstruction.

After the surgery, I was completely horrified at how I looked. At least during the first surgery they had the stitches on the inside. This time they had both stitches and staples on the outside. Now I truly felt like the Bride of Frankenstein. How can anyone ever love me looking like this? I did not want my husband to see me nor did I want to see the look in his eyes when he gazed at my disfigured body. He showed no signs of disgust, but it was what I thought he was feeling. He was just happy I was alive. He did not care what I looked like just as long as I was still around, by his side, to live a long and healthy life. On the ninth day a pick line was inserted so I could be "fed" antibiotics for 6 weeks. At home nursing was provided to check on the pick line and to follow up on my infection. I was very sick for the next 6 weeks due to the antibiotics and was basically bed ridden. When the pick line finally came out, I felt like a new person.

I now can look back on all I've been through, and thirteen months later I can say that I am truly happy to be around. I now know the whole time I thought my asthma was bothering me it was actually angina. As I look back, I can't believe I was in so much denial that it almost killed me. I go to a Heart Support Group at the Heart Center once a month. I have been going since before my surgery, but now I talk to those who I can see are in denial about what is happening. I still get those looks from all the new people that come into Rehab or the Support Group but it doesn't bother me so much any more. I talk to them and try to answer their questions about heart disease. I try to make this event in my life a positive one for others, and also for myself. There are still those occasional days when I feel pain in my chest and it brings all these memories flooding back. But now, I can identify whether the pains are from asthma or acid reflux, which is another problem I live with. Still to this day, I have palpitations, which scare me greatly. But I guess having heart disease is a never-ending battle. I just have longer that I will have to deal with it than most.

Another thing that helps me get through those days of depression, is an organization called Mended Hearts. I joined after having surgery and now I also do Internet visiting for Mended Hearts. I not only get to help others understand the fears they are going through, but it also helps me to see that I am not alone. Heart disease feels like a very lonely disease, but I now find that many share it. I find that more people talk openly over the Internet than in person. Their cries for help are more descriptive and their appreciation is heart warming. I really enjoy helping others understand that they are not alone in their cries for help. Maybe this is the reason I had to have a bypass. Only God knows why, because I sure don't. But let me tell you, I would rather have a bypass anytime than a staph infection; that's for sure.

Since my heart surgery, I also had my gallbladder removed, but otherwise I am doing fine. I am now able to do aerobics at the Heart Center again. I have come a long way physical and emotionally from that dreaded day in May. But now I believe I have a mission. I am here to listen to those who want to tell me their story. Only those who have gone through this really know how these poor souls feel and only we can give them the comfort they seek.

Well that is the end of my story. I hope I did not run on too bad. If you want or need anything else just ask. Thank you for helping others like us. I am sure your book will be a great success.

Good Luck and God Bless.

Angela

*"My message and my preaching were not with wise and persuasive words, but with a demonstration of the Spirit's power, so that your faith might not rest on men's wisdom, but on God's power."*
*1 Corinthians 2:4-5*

*God's word is always the answer to all our questions. His abundant grace is the source of all our needs. Only as time passes can we truly see the work of the master's hand in our lives.*

# Heart Story
## By
## Peter Wenz

In October of 1994, I was a 44-year-old smoker who was somewhat overweight, did not eat the right foods, and exercised very rarely. I had been married for 21 years and we had a healthy two and a half year-old girl that God had placed in our care when she was only 2 days old.

On a Friday night after sleeping for only about two hours, I woke up with this "weird" feeling in my chest. I had no pain, just an unusual sensation. I had my wife call 911 as I got dressed and went out to the street to await the ambulance, which arrived shortly. I was taken to the nearest hospital, where I had all of the routine tests done, and was admitted for observation. After lying around all day Saturday and Sunday, testing resumed on Monday morning with a thallium stress test, which I passed with flying colors. The doctor even remarked that my heart was in "A-one first class condition." On Tuesday, after finding absolutely nothing wrong, I was discharged. I also felt like a fool for causing all the commotion of what seemed to be a false alarm.

Exactly two weeks to the day later, the exact same thing happened. This time I did NOT call 911 again. So I got in the car and told my wife

I was going to the all night drug store to see if I can find something that might help. Halfway there, I realized how stupid that was, made a U-turn and headed back to the hospital again. When I walked in I told them I had this weird sensation in my chest and they of course went into heart attack mode.

I told them to relax, since I had been there two weeks prior and my heart had been checked out, so it must be something else. They ran a bunch of tests anyway, and this time I was discharged early Saturday morning. So I went home and started working in the yard and around the house to get ready for the winter months. About noon I received a call from our family doctor who told me I had to go back to the hospital because they wanted to get to the bottom of what I was experiencing. Of course I didn't want to waste the weekend just lying around, so I asked if I could just check in on Monday morning. The doctor was adamant that I come back that same day. We made a deal that I would go back in that evening after I got all of my work done.

As I found out later on, the EKG they ran after I had been admitted was the first one to show any abnormality of any kind.

They scheduled me for an angiogram first thing Monday morning. At about 6:00 am if I recall correctly. They found that my LAD artery was ninety nine percent blocked, and two others were seventy five percent and fifty percent blocked. The location of the blockage precluded an angioplasty, so the only solution was an emergency bypass.

Unfortunately, the hospital I was in did not do that type of surgery and I would have to be transferred to a different hospital. Knowing that our Pastor was out of town, I asked my wife to call another Pastor friend of mine. Even though he is virtually impossible to get a hold of, he just happened to be home, and was able to meet us at the hospital that I was being transferred too.

Needless to say, that day just flew by. Upon arriving at the hospital, I was informed that the surgery would be about six to eight hours long, and the surgeon who would be doing it already had two scheduled for that day. I would be his third. I remember thinking how he was probably not going to be very happy about doing a third surgery in a row, and I wasn't crazy about it either. Later on I heard that he had in fact requested that my surgery be rescheduled until the next day, but the cardiologist had insisted it be done immediately.

After it was over, the surgeon sat down with my wife and my mother and told them that everything had gone perfectly. He also told them that when he had opened me up, he had found my heart was swollen to twice it's normal size, and that it had already turned completely blue from oxygen deprivation. Yet I had had absolutely no heart damage. He couldn't understand why I had not had a massive heart attack. He also told them that there was no way I could possibly have lived until morning, so it was a good thing they had done the surgery when they did.

I have had an excellent recovery. I quit smoking cigarettes. I improved my diet tremendously. I work out regularly. (I haven't lost any weight though!) God willing, I'll live long enough to walk my little girl down the aisle.

If my heart was that bad, why had I never had a heart attack? Why had I been given two warnings during those two Friday nights? What if our family doctor had not called me up and talked me into checking back in? Why didn't I have a heart attack that Saturday when I was doing heavy physical work while smoking? What if I had been allowed to wait until Monday morning to check in? Then the angiogram would not have been scheduled until Tuesday.

What if the angiogram hadn't taken place until later in the day due to scheduling conflicts? It would then have been too late to transfer me and still receive the operation that same day. Why had it been so easy for my wife to locate the Pastor? What if the surgeon had postponed the surgery until the next day? What if the cardiologist had not insisted on immediate surgery?

The bottom line is that I firmly believe that had it not been for the watchful eye of my Lord Jesus Christ, or one of his angels, I would in likelihood not be here today.

Peter Wenz

*"We live by faith, not by sight"*
*2 Corinthians 5:7*
*She is living it and she is telling it just like it was for her. Misty*
*Craddock is one of the most informed heart patients I have spoken*
*with. She is eager for knowledge of her own care, as well as the*
*care of others. Misty relates to me that she has accepted her situa-*
*tion and acts on it immediately whenever the need arises. Her atti-*
*tude now, as compared to when she was experiencing her diagnosis*
*and treatments, has entirely changed. Misty is a survivor and keeps*
*abreast of the latest in research and available treatment. There is*
*LIFE with heart disease.*

# Misty Craddock
# Her Story

I read everything I could get my hands on after I had surgery. I even ordered medical books from Majors Bookstore out of Houston, Texas. That cost me a lot of money. I only wish that I'd had the wonder of the Internet way back then. I have learned so much over the years about coronary artery disease. In 1986, when I first got sick and had to have surgery, I had no idea what to expect, and no one to talk to. I did attend rehab, but all the other patients were much older than I was, so I never felt like I belonged there. By the time I had symptoms, the CAD was already severe, with total occlusion of the LAD & the RCA, with high-grade stenosis in several places in the circumflex. It was at this time, that I learned I also had a genetic hyperlipidemia, which by the way, no one else in my immediate family has. I did not and still do not, have a weight problem. I did however, smoke cigarettes.

After the triple bypass, I did very well for eight and one half years before the angina reappeared.

The moment it did, I knew what had happened and my heart sunk to my feet. I tried to deny the facts, but progressively got worse over the next few months. I finally went to my cardiologist, who performed a thallium stress test, which, of course, showed multiple ischemic areas. An angiogram showed that all of my native coronary arteries were totally occluded and that one of the mammary artery grafts was totally occluded, and the other mammary was approximately eighty percent blocked. The only graft still totally patent was the vein graft to the RCA, although there were areas of disease in the distal part of the PDA. With these findings, the best treatment for me would be another CABG. The cardiac surgeon would not perform the surgery, due to the fact that in the previous bypass surgery, the surgeons had crossed the mammary arteries beneath my sternum and they had adhered very firmly to the underside of the sternum, prohibiting re-entry through the sternum for another surgery. So my cardiologist treated me medically with more and more medicines adding to the ever-growing number, until even those ceased to help me very much. From stable angina, I gradually progressed to unstable angina associated with even dreams, sad movies, or just about any type of emotional surge. It happened walking to the mailbox, in the grocery store, washing my hair—you get the picture.

In 1997, the disease process had progressed to the point that either I had to have redo bypass surgery, or have a massive MI that the doctors assured me I could not survive as it would involve the entire left ventricle. There happened to be a fairly new cardiovascular surgeon here that my doctor showed the new angiogram films to. Well, this surgeon felt challenged by the case, and asked me if he could try to come up with some way to help me, which was fine by me, of course. His solution was to do a minicab to bypass the totally blocked mammary, followed four months later by a left thoracotomy incision to reach the ninety percent blocked mammary artery. He tried to reach the vein graft to the RCA, because that had developed disease of three eighty to ninety five percent blockages. He was unable to reach it far enough down to bypass, so he just left it as it was, with the notion that it could be opened later with PTCA if I continued to have angina. By the way, this surgery was at least three times as painful as the very first one through the sternum! I again attended rehab and still had angina, which severely dampened my hopes of the total angina relief achieved from the first CABG eleven years previously.

After I completed rehab, my cardiologist performed another angiogram with the intention of opening the vein graft to the RCA with angioplasty and possibly a stent. Well, the graft was found to be totally closed off, so he did nothing to it. However, he also found a new ninety five percent blockage near the bypassed area of the last mammary bypass performed four months previously, which he was able to balloon open, but was, too near a branch to put a stent into it. I continue to have exertion angina, but nowhere nearly as severe as before and nothing; I cannot live with. My blood pressure is very well controlled on Diovan HCT and my lipid levels are excellent now. I also have PVD for which bilateral iliac angioplasties were done a few months after my first CABG, and then an aorta-femoral endarterectomy was done in 1992, which helped me tremendously to walk farther without as much pain.

I'm sorry this is so long, but this is what I've had since 1986. I feel I'm doing very well, and know my heart, and body well. I will fight this disease process every step of the way! I will NEVER give up the good fight and will go out kicking and yelling!

You asked about the emotional aspect, and if I'm to be totally honest, it has kicked the stuffing out of me many times. I still get scared, and your psychologist friend said it all with the comment about "night terrors." Night is the worst time for me. That's when I ponder my future, when I feel the most vulnerable, when I'm afraid to go to sleep, for fear of not waking up. You see, I've developed a morbid fear of death and can, at times, work myself into a state of panic. I refuse to take any type of mood altering drugs such as antidepressants, tranquilizers, or sleeping pills, due to an inner hang up of needing to feel in control at all times and to be able to see what comes next. I have periods of depression if I allow myself to dwell too much on all this, so

I attempt to look on the bright side. With the modern technologies available today to fight this disease, and the new ones on the horizon, my own role is taking care of my health, and in educating myself because I feel that knowledge is power in this fight.

I do want to add that I did not stop smoking after the first CABG, nor were we ever able to get my lipids under good enough control, both of which might have contributed to the occlusion of my grafts so soon after bypass. This time around I expect them to remain open for a lot longer. I have corrected every risk factor under my control. I do worry about going through menopause and losing that "protective" estrogen.

Misty Craddock

*A dramatic story filled with the power of God, to provide HOPE in a situation that appears hopeless. We all must remember that where there is LIFE, there is hope. Nothing is impossible with God. He is forever present to sustain us, carry us in our darkest hours if we only believe and trust in him.*

*"Blessed is he who has regard for the weak; the Lord delivers him in times of trouble. The Lord will protect him and preserve his life; he will bless him in the land and not surrender him to the desires of his foes. The Lord will sustain him on his sickbed and restore him from his bed of illness."*
*Psalm 41:1-3*

# Heart Transplant Experience
## by
## Nancy Williams

In 1986, at the age of 46, I had bypass surgery and went on with my stressful life as if nothing had even been wrong.

In 1991, I had another full-blown heart attack. When I woke up in the intensive care unit the next day, I was shocked when the doctor told me there was nothing that could be done except a heart transplant. I stupidly thought that he would do everything necessary when the time came that I would need the transplant. I was so wrong. He never referred me to an appropriate hospital for evaluation to be put on a transplant list. For over a year he allowed me to just grow weaker and weaker. My ejection fraction was fourteen percent. I lost a tremendous amount of weight. Finally, in September, I called the general practitioner that had been taking care of me and asked for another opinion. This time I took my mugga scan and echo cardiogram to the new doctor in October of 1992.

His first question was how did I walk into his office? His second question was how long had I been on the transplant list. I asked a silly question. "What list?" Needless to say, he was on the phone to UPMC in Pittsburgh. Within days, I was scheduled for evaluation the third week in November. My first thought was that I had already wasted a year and my time was running out. Even if I did make the list I would never live long enough to get a heart. I was nearly right. On December 6, 1992, I called the ambulance. I was filling with fluid and couldn't breathe. I was put into ICU on Debutimin, but by now I was almost too weak to walk. Around the 14th,I had another heart attack.

I had a living will that said "No artificial life supports." I was ready to die. I did not want to be a vegetable being kept alive. My loving partner overrode my wishes because the doctor explained that as long as I was on the list, there was hope. If they took me off the list, they would let me go. Each Friday, it is my understanding that decisions are made regarding who stays on the list. Someone must have put up a fight to keep me on it, because they told George that if I continued to fail they would take me off the list and life support and let me go. This was told to him Friday, the 18th. He left the hospital so he could call our families and prepare them for what might happen.

At 2:00 a.m., my doctor came into my room removed the respirator and informed me that they had a heart for me. They then brought a portable phone into my room for me to call George and my son. You can imagine the shock he had hearing my voice.

I went into surgery at 9:00 a.m., and came out close to 3:00 p.m. There was a leak in one of the arteries so I was taken back into surgery and did not come out until 2:00 a.m. the following morning. Because I was so weak when I received the heart, I was in the hospital until January 14th. My return to health was slow but steady.

In the first part one of my story I told you about how the cardiologist was allowing me to die by not helping me to get on the transplant list. From August of 1991 until I changed doctors in October of 1992, I was putting my affairs in order. Getting ready to die. I had a will made out and was going through all of my file folders so that my family would be able to find everything they would need upon my death. I was trying to make it easy for them.

The most important thing I did was to make a living will. In 1991 a living will had not been tested in court so my living will was more about my wishes than it was about any legal document that the doctors or my family could truly rely on. Just so you can understand why my living will was written the way it was, I have to go back to the death of both of my parents. My father had a heart attack and a stroke in May of 1973. He seemed to be slowly improving when he had an aneurysm in September of the same year. I do not remember if my Mother was ever asked about artificial life supports but even if she had, she would have adamantly turned them down. As it was he lived from Sunday until Thursday. At times, I felt he could hear us but he just went deeper and deeper in a coma.

I had just returned to work, when my mother, who had previously had at least four heart attacks that put her in the hospital over 18 years, had a stroke. The stroke affected the part of her brain that controlled reasoning and logic. They sent her home from the hospital even though she kept getting lost and confused. She lived alone. I had my own business and I tried to get twenty four-hour help for her. She fired them as fast as I could hire them. She had always trusted me now she hung up notes telling me to leave her groceries and get out. Well, to make a long story, as short as, possible she went to a personal care home when I was put back into the hospital for bypass surgery in October of 1986. While she was in that personal care home she had another stroke and was taken to a hospital where a doctor did not know her or her family. He had only minutes to decide whether to put her on a respirator. He chose to do that. For days, I sat next to her bed watching that machine breathe for her. She was not alive. I made a terrible mistake. Her feet were cold and I wanted to put a pair of socks on them. When I lifted the sheet, she was black to the waist. I screamed at the doctor to get her off of that machine, but he legally could not. I had no legal recourse unless I wanted to go to court and this could take months. The doctor agreed with me, but his hands were tied. Our only hope was that her weak heart would give out soon. It did after about a week.

Now that leads me to my part of the story. I wrote a living will. I said, "No artificial life supports." My family and George knew I meant it even though it might not hold up in court. I was ready to die. In November of 1992, I was finally told that I had been put on the transplant list. That meant absolutely nothing to me. I knew about how wonderful a man from my church was doing and that is what helped me to decide to go through the evaluation to be put on the list, but by now I was too weak to even care. On December 6th, when I called the ambulance to take me to the hospital, I really went there to die. I felt that there was so little hope. I was even more depressed when I was put into a room next to a man that had already been there for six months.

About a week after I arrived in the hospital I had a massive heart attack. My bowels let go. I begged the doctor to give me something to stop the pain. They kept trying to put an oxygen mask on me and I kept ripping it off. Oxygen does not help when your lungs are filled with fluid. I know that a respirator was suggested and I was awake enough to say NO. But, my living will said the following. "If I am unable to make decisions for myself then George can make them for me."

The next thing I remember was waking up in intensive care on a respirator. And I was angry! I was later told that, as soon as the doctor read my living will, he gave me a shot of morphine. He then turned to George and said, "Now she cannot make decisions for herself. Her heart is so weak that if I give her more drugs it may stop and we will not be able to start it again." "SHE IS ON THE TRANSPLANT LIST AND THERE IS STILL HOPE!"

George agreed under the condition that if I was taken off the list and all hope of a transplant was gone, then I would also be taken off the respirator. Every time he came into my room and I was even slightly awake I would make him give me the clipboard with one sheet of paper on it and a pen. I can remember writing the following things on that piece of paper. I always print in capitals. "TAKE ME OFF THIS THING," "YOU AND THE DOCTORS ARE NOT LISTENING TO ME. GET MY DOCTORS," "CAN'T THEY LET ME GO EASY?"

I was so drugged that I would keep turning that clipboard until George would hold it still, but I knew what I did not want. I did not want artificial life supports.

Patiently, George would explain to me. "Nancy, you are still on the list and as long as you are on the list there is still hope. Do you understand me?" A few days went by and I must have been holding my own because they took me off the respirator. When they did that my doctors stood at my bed and said in no uncertain terms that they would not put it back in unless I gave my permission verbally right then. He even used tough love. He almost shouted at me that he was leaving for the night and he did not want to be called out of his sleep. I was still on the list. Did I understand that there was still hope? I nodded each time. Yes, I understood but I was so tired. It would be so much easier if they would just let me go.

There was George, with at least a two-day beard. How much I hurt for him and my son. They were watching me die. Wouldn't it just be easier for everyone if I could just go to sleep?

But, they wanted an answer NOW. With tears in my eyes I looked at George and told him I did not know what to say. He told me to say yes. In a very low voice going against everything that I thought was right, I said yes. Then I asked George if I had done the right thing. He smiled and said yes.

I wasn't off the respirator very long when I crashed again and had to be put back on. I can remember them shouting, "Nancy swallow!" "Nancy swallow!"

Every Friday the transplant decisions are made. Who gets on the list, and who stays on the list?

Friday night around 8 p.m., while I was still on the respirator, my doctors took George into a small private room next to the CC ICU unit and told him that I was on the list on an hour by hour basis. If my other organs continued to fail, they would take me off the respirator and let me go. Someone had fought to keep me on that list. George left the hospital shortly after visiting hours so that he could go home and call both of our families. He fully intended to get a shower, shave get some much needed sleep and be back at the hospital early Saturday. He really felt that the doctors were just trying to give him time to face my possible death.

At 2:00 a.m., just hours after George left, they came into my room, reversed the drug that was keeping me sleeping, took out the respirator and told me that a heart had come in.

George had fallen asleep on the sofa. No shower, no shave. And most of all no phone calls from the transplant team. They had told me at 2:00 a.m., that they would get in touch with my family, meaning my son and George. We only lived twenty minutes from the hospital. No one came. The surgery was scheduled for 9:00 a.m. Saturday morning December 19, 1992 and I was alone. My male nurse finally brought me a portable phone at about 6:00 a.m. Can you even imagine what the following words did to George, "Where are you?" They told me at 2:00 a.m., that they have a heart for me and I am going into surgery?" I do not even remember his reply.

The first thing I remember, after that, was someone tearing the page off the daily calendar and reading the words, Thursday December 23rd. I have been so blessed because I have not had any rejection. My quality of life is great. I only wish that each person in this world could understand how important it is to say and do each thing every day as if it was to be his or her last day on earth. What a wonderful world this would be.

God! What a beautiful Christmas present I had been given. I was really going to live. Now it was up to me. It is my job to protect the gift that was given to me and do everything I can to give something back. I keep asking myself. Why am I here?

Was it because a 52-year-old man put an organ donor sticker on his license? Was it because his family made a very painful decision? Was it because my doctors fought to keep me on the transplant list after probably saving my life a few times for a week? Was it because George made the decision to override my living will? Was it because I did not know how to say NO? I have never been able to say that word to anyone. Was it because I was in one of the best hospitals and had one of the best surgeons in the country?

Was it because God wanted me here? Maybe it is all of those reasons but all along the way no one let me give up hope.

Now here is a postscript to my story. When I came out of surgery and off the respirator I asked George, my wonderful partner, "If you could go anywhere in the world where would you like to go?" His answer was Australia. So, in March of this year, we took a wonderful trip. We flew to Los Angeles on March 13, and stayed overnight and spent the day with my cousin. We then boarded a plane and flew twelve hours to Auckland, New Zealand. From there we boarded a cruise ship that stopped at eight ports in New Zealand, Hobart and Australia. When we got off the ship in Sydney, we spent two nights there before we took a thirteen hours flight back to LAX. We again spent the night before our five-hour flight home. We arrived back April 1st. It was a wonderful experience and I know that I helped to fulfill George's dream. So you see wonderful things do happen. The down side of this is that this may be the last very long trip we take. George has asbestosis (from working around asbestos at his job) and also emphysema. This trip was very hard on him but it did not spoil it in any way. I really believe that he is the reason that God kept me here.

God Bless all of the caregivers out there and God bless all of you that are waiting.

Nancy Williams

*Read the childhood memories that can be used to support and encourage children not to fear, as told by Linda of her surgery.*

*"Let the little children come to me, and do not hinder then, for the kingdom of heaven belongs to such as these."*
*Jesus said in Matthew 19: 13*

# Atrial Septial Defect
## By
## Linda Hussey, R.N.

24 November 1999

In 1961, at the age of four, I had open-heart surgery. I was born with Atrial Septial Defect. My mother was a Registered Nurse. Working in Key West, Florida at the time and met a heart surgeon who had just gotten a promotion to be head of cardiology at a larger hospital in New York. Mom really trusted him, this was back then heart surgery was a scary surgery. She quit her job and followed him to New York so he could operate on me. She was without a job, and was fortunate that he did not charge her for the surgery. I don't remember much about it except that I was always sick prior to surgery. I was always hospitalized with pneumonia and couldn't run with other kids, etc. Once in the hospital, I remember trying to run away, I packed my overnight case with my favorite toys and while clad in pjs, I managed to get to an elevator and down to the 1st floor where some nurses coming on duty stopped me. I guess I was scared!

I remember waking up after the surgery and being in this big plastic monster O2 tent. I screamed, and I remember all the needles and tubes sticking in me. When it was time to pull the tubes on either side of me,

I screamed for my mom to do it, and they did let her assist because I screamed so much.

After the surgery, I remember that I couldn't wait till I could play with the other kids—running, etc. and my amazement when I was allowed too. Growing up after the surgery was really uneventful. I got checked every two years, and had to take antibiotics for dental work.

When I was thirteen, I developed pneumonia, strep throat, and mono all at the same time and my heart specialist was afraid my surgery was not holding up. I had a heart catherization, which I loved. I watched the screen and asked more questions than they wanted to answer, but they did! The results were good, with my heart with the exception, of a murmur.

Now that I'm the tender age of 42, I have three kids that I delivered. No, I didn't adopt each time—they had a cardiologist on call in case something happened. But each time I never saw him! I still follow up with my doctor every two years. I just went in September and had an echogram, and everything is still okay. Life is just fine! Once, when I was in college and doing my clinical, I helped out in the emergency room as a student and ran into a scared 13 year old who was having problems with her heart and she was being admitted for yes, you guessed it, heart surgery. I went to her and said, "Hey, I look pretty healthy ugh?" and she said "yeah why?" Then I told my story and she didn't seem quite so scared.

Linda Hussey R.N.

*Mr. Driver gives the credit up front for his recovery. He quoted to me that he was not afraid because the Lord had always told him he would never forsake him. He trusted what the Lord said and just did it.*

*"For the Lord thy God is a merciful God; he will not forsake thee, neither destroy thee, nor forget the covenant of thy fathers which he swore unto them."*
*Deuteronomy: 4 31*

# Coronary Artery Bypass Grafts
## BY
## William C. Driver

First, I have to say that I have a deep belief in God and I give him all the credit for my recovery.

For about six months, I had been having chest pain and was taking Nitrostat like it was candy. I am 73 years old, and a member of my home church Family Bible Church in Oak Harbor, Washington. Having experienced a great deal of chest pain that was making me short of breath, I knew it was a matter of time until I had to have something done.

I also have sleep apnea and use a C Path machine to help me sleep. It works wonders for me to be able to get a good night sleep.

One day, I was riding in my truck and decided to go to my doctor's office to get a refill on my Nitrostat prescription. My regular doctor was not in and his assistant decided to check me over before writing me a new prescription. He came back in and told me he wasn't going to write a new prescription that I was going to the hospital to be checked in. It was time to make a decision to have something done.

My doctor explained to me what had to be done by showing me pictures of the heart and exactly what he was going to do. That helped to relieve my fears a lot. I knew I couldn't live like I was.

On April 21, 1999, I was going to surgery for bypass. I was given seven bypasses in surgery. My wife June was with me all the time. She stayed with me constantly and even slept on a cot in my room.

On the day of the surgery I asked for the Chaplin to come to the surgery area and read to me out loud the 23rd Psalm. I then turned it over to the Lord because he said in his word that He would never leave me or forsake me and I trusted Him to do what he said. So the Lord and I went to surgery. I went through the surgery fine, but had problems later with my heart rate being too slow.

They used the paddles on me to shock my heart back to rhythm and when they touched me with those electrical paddles I yelled "OH, LORD" out loud. The Lord came through. I was given a pacemaker to help my heart to beat normal.

I have to admit that I went through a lot of depression after my heart surgery and was put on medication to control it. I had a lot of fears, but I was determined to just turn it over to the Lord and let him take care of me. My wife June and I are very close and stay very active. I a.m. a swimmer and swim at least three times a week. We go to the senior citizen meetings and play pinochle on Tuesday and Fridays.

I no longer take the depression medication, and I have to say that I give all the Glory to God for my recovery and continued progress. Looking back on it all, I can truly say that God was looking out after me. If I had called to get the prescription refilled instead of going to the office where the doctor insisted on checking me out I don't know what would have happened. I thank God daily and give him all the glory.

This is my story, and I hope it serves to help anyone who reads it and will trust in the Lord for all, their needs.

William C. Driver
Washington

*Colette's, new diagnosis of heart disease is told by her, in a straight forward, account of her physical and emotional devastation she experienced upon diagnosis. Her ability to cope with her diagnosis, and with an exciting new awakening. of being able to help others in a similar situations. Thank you Colette for your honest and self-revealing experience that had to be difficult to relive in such a poignant way.*

*"Have I not commanded you? Be strong and courageous. Do not be terrified; do not be discouraged, for the Lord your God will be with you wherever you go."*
*Joshua 1:9*

# Coronary Artery Bypass Graft
# Colette's Experience

24 November 1999

The tingling started on one of those beautiful days in May. You know the type, the birds are singing, and the sweet smell of new blossoms hangs in the air?

"Funny," I thought. "I've never had this tingling in the ring and little finger of my left hand before. I must have hit my elbow." But the tingling continued, blinking off and on like a bad light bulb. It bothered me, but I dismissed it.

A couple of weeks later, I began to experience other tingling in my back and chest—a funny, strange tingle that wasn't pleasant, but which lasted only a few seconds nothing more. I came to dread these new tingles. They weren't pleasant; in fact they were becoming downright scary! Somewhat like a bolt of lightning and a buzz hitting all at once. Still, I thought I must have a nerve problem with my back. How easily I shrugged it all off, even with the episodes becoming more and more frequent.

I shrugged off other symptoms too. My gums were bleeding profusely. My lower jaws ached (Well, I'd always had TMJ!) and I was losing weight at a tremendous rate (visions of the big "C" word danced in my head). I didn't know my heart had started to work overtime!

On Friday, May 21, 1999, I enjoyed a late, but wonderful dinner of steak, baked potato with butter, yellow squash, green bean casserole and watermelon (Many heart attacks occur after a good meal!) I fell asleep, only to awaken at around 12:30a.m. with what I thought was the worst heartburn I'd ever experienced. It was a crushing, difficult-to-breathe heartburn. I couldn't find a good position to lay because I was so uncomfortable.

So what did I do? You guessed it! Pepcid AC to the rescue! But, it didn't work. Although, I had guessed what was wrong, I wouldn't admit it even to myself. Heart attack! No! Not me! I was only 49 years old! My dad had a heart attack several years before due to stress, but his symptoms hadn't been similar to this. He'd just had a couple fainting spells. His heart had worked out new pathways on its own; so nothing was done.

But I had a history of hypertension and high cholesterol. Drugs I'd tried hadn't worked to lower my cholesterol; neither had diet. I was at risk more than most people and I was writhing in pain. But, did I wake anyone in my household up? Of course not! The Pepcid AC hadn't worked, so I decided to take an aspirin just in case. I'd seen TV commercials advising chewing an aspirin at the first sign of heart attack, but I was loathe to chew it so I swallowed one with a glass of hot water.

Afterward, I became nauseated and vomited. I felt better. And I went back to sleep, unaware that I'd just experienced my first heart attack.

The weekend passed uneventfully, with just a few minor episodes of those awful tingles in my back and chest. I was back to normal! But, just in case, I started to carry a bottle of aspirin in my purse. That Monday I ran to the store for a couple items and during the drive the tingling returned with a vengeance. Then the 'heartburn' struck. I staggered inside the store, turned around and got back into my car. It was a beautiful, sun-drenched day in Florida and I always carry a bottle of water with me. The water was hot from sitting in the car and I took my aspirin once again with hot water. The pain eased and I re-entered the store. By the time I reached the checkout lanes I was in pain again, gasping for breath. A hospital sat right across the street, so I got back into my car and drove to the emergency room. Big mistake! Don't ever, ever drive if you think you're having a heart attack!

I parked outside the emergency room but I didn't go in. Why? I thought I'd feel foolish if it just turned out to be heartburn after all! Later, I discovered that most heart attack victims that die do so feeling afraid of looking 'foolish' and are found usually clutching a package of Tums.

The pain abated, and I drove home without going inside. I wasn't aware that I'd just had my second heart attack.

I had an appointment with my internist the following day. Not because of my symptoms, but to get a prescription filled. His physician assistant took care of me, and on my way out, I casually mentioned my severe 'heartburn'—Yep, casually!

Before I knew it, I was having an EKG. The physicians assistant felt there was something wrong with it and had the nurse refer me to a local cardiologist, while scheduling me for a recheck in one week.

Well, the cardiologist's office had not yet called to schedule my appointment when I reappeared for my recheck with my Internist. As he reviewed my previous EKG he stated "Women's EKG's are very hard to read. I think you have Gastric Reflux Disease with a possible Hiatus Hernia. Your glucose level is also up, so I'd like to additional blood work to rule out diabetes."

Oh, how I wanted to believe him! In fact, he further stated that "Women absolutely don't ever have symptoms of heartburn with their heart attacks." No pun intended, but as much as I wanted to believe him I knew in my heart that he was wrong. I'd gotten on the Internet and discovered a myriad of heart attack symptoms all relating to my episodes. They included heartburn in women and elevated glucose levels after a major trauma to the body such as a heart attack.

In spite of my Internet research results, I honestly wanted to believe my internist. So when the cardiologist's office finally scheduled my appointment, I was in no hurry. I was scheduled for a Cardiolite Stress Test the following week.

I arrived at the hospital with plenty of time to spare, shaking inside. I knew I would be injected with a chemical that would put my heart under stress as if I was on a treadmill. The solution would also contain radioactive isotopes. It was a two-day test, with the heart being under stress the first day and the heart at rest (no chemicals) the second. I was terrified. My dad had had a similar test two years previous (a Thallium Induced Stress Test), and told me that he'd had severe angina during the test. The hospital itself didn't help when they asked me to sign a release stating that the test might result in cardiac arrest, coma or death. It's a standard release, but I couldn't handle reading it. All I saw, were those words, cardiac arrest, coma, or death.

As I was about to sign the paper, I noticed the cardiologist performing the test was not my doctor. I questioned this, and was told my doctor was scheduled at another hospital and this doctor would be taking his place. What a perfect excuse! I jumped at it.

"I want my own doctor, not just anyone!" This was my one chance to run out of there, and I was terrified enough to go with it—and I mean run in the literal sense! I ran out of the hospital, leaving the nurses to call my doctor's nurse to have the test rescheduled. It was the worst mistake of my life, which I'll tell you about later on.

Two more weeks passed before the test was rescheduled. I was still having minor heartburn and tingling. Sometimes, it was hard to breathe. And, I was so very, very tired and cold. It was late May in Florida, hot and humid, and I was cold. I was also losing weight rapidly, and for the first time in years I could eat anything I wanted to eat and still lose, unaware that this was because my heart was working far too hard. I started to eat a heart-healthy portion of oatmeal every morning, just in case it could still help lower my cholesterol.

I was trying to do everything right, too late. I still hadn't told my family or friends anything at this point. I merely showed up at the hospital for the rescheduled Cardiolite Stress Test. I was still absolutely terrified. I still wanted to believe my internist-that it wasn't my heart. But, I showed up for the test, so scared that I was crying hysterically. When my doctor showed up, an IV solution was started in my arm. The doctor was very kind, patient and comforting, as was the radiologist. I felt pressure in my chest during the test, but it was over within a few minutes. I often wonder how many other cardiac patients become hysterical during these tests!

Before he left, my doctor turned to me and said, "You have a very serious problem in the left front part of your heart." "Until we finish the test and I see you in my office, do NOT lift anything at all or lift your arms above your head."

Can you imagine my feelings when he said this? If anyone ever needed a major tranquilizer, it's me! Still, I refused to believe this was happening to me! Oh, Not me, not my HEART. No!

I think the hardest part of the two-day test was lying still under the nuclear machine. It was like a huge CAT scan machine, and it took x-rays for about an hour. The following day was easier. It is a ten-minute scan without medication, showing my heart at rest.

I thought, with the test over, that I was home free. My parents were away on vacation and I was at their house watching the cat, when my cell phone rang that afternoon. "The doctor would like to see you in his office as soon as you can get here," the nurse stated.

Now, we've all seen on TV how the doctors will call patients in to give them bad news. I thought it could never happen to me, but it did, in just that way. As soon as I entered the office, I was ushered past the other patients into a private office. My doctor told me that the stress test confirmed a blockage in the left main part of my heart, the most dangerous place to have something wrong. He wanted me in the hospital immediately, that evening, for an angiogram the following morning.

My family didn't even know where I was! I called my 25-year-old son to go with me. I was so frightened that I was on the verge of a breakdown.

And, break down I did! I shook, I cried, I cringed. I refused an IV; later the head nurse talked me into it. I was placed on a portable monitor. I cried some more. I refused to sleep, afraid that I might die in my sleep, and sat up in a chair all night long. As morning approached, I called my son to come get me. I couldn't go through with the angiogram. I don't know what I was more afraid of the angiogram itself or hearing the results. I just know that I convinced myself that I would die if I had the test. I left the hospital, AMA—against medical advice.

The cardiologist called me at home He called my internist, who also called me at home. Both office nurses called me at home. All of them begged and pleaded with me to return to the hospital. I refused. I told myself that if God wanted to take me, I'd go naturally when it was my time and not during a test. Oh, how stupid I was!

A few nights later, I had no choice. I'd been prescribed a Nitro patch to wear, along with Nitro pills with instructions to wear the patch during the day only. The Nitro pills were to be taken at the first sign of angina—one pill, wait for 5 minutes. Then, take another pill if still experiencing symptoms of pain. Wait another 5 minutes. If I needed a third pill, I was to go by ambulance to the nearest ER.

That day, I disregarded all of my doctor's instructions regarding lifting or using my arms. I washed windows and washed my car. I trimmed a bush outside. I began to experience angina, and I ended up being rushed to ER around 9 p.m. that night.

The choice is made for me now. I knew this was serious and I began to accept that my heart needed help. An IV was started in the ambulance. I was told that since it was started in an "non-sterile environment," that I'd receive another IV as soon as I was admitted to the hospital.

That didn't happen. No one replaced that IV, not that day or in the days to follow. I was admitted to ICU; and heparin a blood thinner, was started and an angiogram scheduled for the following morning. No one told me that this hospital was only licensed to perform angiograms and NOT angioplasty or heart surgery. I later found out that this particular hospital was required to perform a certain number of angiograms prior to being licensed for any type of surgery. I'd had no choice. The ambulance took me to the nearest hospital as was their protocol.

The following morning, the angiogram was performed. I was given a light sedative. A catheter was inserted through an incision in my right femoral artery and threaded up into my heart where a dye was injected. I watched the procedure on video next to me, but I didn't know what to look for. I didn't feel much of anything except when the catheter was inside my left ventricle. At that point, I felt flushed and my heart felt 'fluttery'. This only lasted a few seconds. Then, I was given a copy of a 'picture' of my heart and the blockage found. A ninety percent to ninety five percent blockage in the LAD, (left anterior descending artery). It looked so tiny on the picture! How, I wondered, could something so tiny be so serious?

Following the angiogram, I was to be transferred by ambulance to a hospital on the other side of town, where a PTCA—balloon angioplasty with a stent was performed. The doctor decided to leave the catheter in my femoral artery so that another wouldn't need to be inserted during the next procedure. I was forbidden to move and had to lay flat in the hospital bed because of the catheter in my leg. I had to eat lying flat on my back, and use a bedpan, etc. It was horrible! But, at least by this time, I was more accepting of my fate. Besides, I couldn't run out of there if I'd wanted too!

By the following morning, more than 24 hours had passed with the catheter still in my leg. I was having terrible spasms in my back, arms and legs. I wanted to brush my teeth and wash up, but I wasn't allowed to move. Finally, I was transferred by ambulance to the other hospital where it was discovered I was now running a fever. Five more hours passed until it was determined that the PTCA could not be performed. My fever raged and my muscles were in spasms. The catheter was removed, but I still had to lay flat another 4 hours.

By this time, I was in absolute agony. I was taken to a room on the cardiac floor, hooked to monitors and on constant heparin, while an infectious disease control specialist was called in. One look at the IV in my arm, (the IV that had been started in the ambulance) and the redness and puffiness that surrounded it told him that this was the infection site. The IV was finally removed and replaced in another site. Vancomycin, an IV antibiotic was started. I remained on Heparin and Vancomycin for a week, since the PTCA could not be performed on a patient running a fever. I needed to be fever free for 24 hours, and my temperature kept spiking. While I begged to go home, the nurses started referring to me as "The walking dead woman in 323." Once again, I was forbidden to use my arms or to lift them above my head. That meant no showers, and no hair washing. I felt dirty and depressed. I cried constantly and still had not slept! My eyes were sunken and had deep blue circles underneath, and I continued to beg to go home. When sedatives were offered, I'd scream at the nurses "Is that what you do, you drug the patients into submission to make your job easier?" I was the worst patient on this earth!

Finally, the big day arrived. I hadn't wanted anyone at the hospital with me, but my parents and my son showed up anyway. My cardiologist arrived and explained to me that the PTCA procedure would only take about twenty minutes. First, a catheter would once again be placed in my femoral artery (in the upper thigh near my crotch), and a fine wire would be threaded up into my heart, as in the angiogram, I'd had. The blockage would be opened with a balloon and a stent placed in the blockage to hold the artery open. A stent is a similar to a tiny spring. The wire would be withdrawn after the stent was placed and tissue would grow around the stent, holding it in place.

He added that he had not had a stent failure resulting in bypass surgery during the past 2 1/2 years, but an emergency team would be standing by, just in case I needed a single bypass. I didn't want to sign the consent form for emergency bypass surgery, but I was afraid not too. It would be just my luck to be his first failure!

I was wheeled to a small operating room and lightly sedated. I knew everything that was happening, but I didn't care and it seemed that within minutes the procedure was over. The doctor stood up, walked to a video room and spoke with the technicians a few minutes. Then, he calmly returned to me and said, "I'm sorry, the stent failed to hold and is moving. You will need the emergency bypass after all."

I remember thinking "Oh, just my luck." I was afraid, yet calm. I was wheeled to a holding area and my son was called in. I asked him to call his father and brother and I kissed him goodbye. Suddenly, a team ran into the room and started wheeling me down the hall, with the guy at the head of my gurney shouting orders and another climbing onto the end of my bed. I remember thinking "Wow!" This is just like on ER, the television show! I wonder when they're going to put me out. Eight hours later, I was awakened by the Open Heart ICU nurse. The bypass was over. The surgeon, whom I later discovered had been the one shouting orders at the head of my gurney, appeared briefly and said, "Hi, I'm the guy who saved your life!" At first I thought he was being just a little too smug. Later I discovered he was right. I'd been dying on the table. He explained he'd ended up performing a triple bypass.

"Triple!" I screamed (or thought I screamed-I was later told I'd whispered a result of being on a respirator for two hours following surgery). "My doctor promised I'd only need a SINGLE bypass!" As if it made a difference! But, it did to me. The surgeon explained that my stent had kept moving and ripped my artery. That every time he touched my heart tissue, it more or less dissolved in his fingers, due to the stent, and resulted in a triple bypass for a single blockage.

Later, through much Internet research, and the opinions of several neurologists and cardiologists, I discovered that stents normally aren't used in a LAD artery to begin with! It's a very dangerous place to place a stent. Perhaps my cardiologist hadn't fully expanded the stent because of its location. I wondered had he fully expanded the stent. My heart might have been deprived of blood too long and gone into full cardiac arrest. Because stents are designed to NOT move once fully expanded and in place!

As a result, the saphenous vein in my left thigh was used, resulting in permanent nerve damage, nerve pain and total numbness of the leg below the knee. I needed two blood transfusions, post-op. I had a long scar going down the middle of my chest, from the neck to mid-abdomen. I remained on IV fluids and Vancomycin, an antibiotic for another week, for fear the infection from that first IV would return and invade my heart. All this is due to a stent that wasn't supposed to move but did. I'm lucky, though! I did everything wrong—yet I'm alive. I've dedicated the rest of my life to helping others facing heart surgery. I beg them to NOT follow my example! Don't be too afraid of the tests or the surgery. Without them, I wouldn't be here. Investigate your doctor's credentials, get second or third opinions. Don't be an uninformed victim of hospital or doctor error, like I was. Research your options, find the best surgeons in your area and follow their instructions. It may save your life.

Collette

*Jay had bypass surgery complicated by sleep apnea. His experience is dramatic and yet uplifting in every detail. He is an experienced medical professional and still his symptoms eluded him.*

# Jay's Heart Experience

Who would of thought that after assessing hundreds of heart attack patients and doing CPR more times than I would like to remember, I could not diagnose my own chest pains. Approximately two years after I was diagnosed with a Hiatal Hernia, I began to have mid-sternum pain, which I attributed to the hiatal hernia. I shrugged it off, missing the first symptom of chest pains. About six months later, I began to have jaw pain. I have false teeth, and I attributed it too improper fitting dentures, the second symptom, (What an idiot?). I was backpacking with my ex-wife Cheryl, and I began to have severe left arm pain, bingo, I figured it out. Did I go to the hospital? No, I finished the backpacking trip and went to see a cardiologist the following day.

The first thing the cardiologist did was order, a stress test to be done on me. This lasted all of 11 seconds before he told me to get off. The doctor told me I needed to get an angiogram immediately. Unfortunately, I told him he would have to wait a week. I needed to get all my affairs in order. I promised I would not think about work or work during that week. At the time, I was President of a fairly large ambulance company. The following week my angiogram showed a ninety seven percent blockage of the widow maker. Because I worked out with weights very hard, the collateral blood flow kept me alive. It was determined I needed a triple bypass. Then my cardiologist came in the room with the good news, bad news routine. The bad news, the triple bypass—the good news, I was alive.

My doctor asked me if I had a cardiac surgeon, which of course I did not. He proceeded to look out into the hallway and asked a doctor to come in. He explained to the cardiac surgeon what I needed and said he would handle it if I wanted him to do the job. If you recall, I mentioned I ran an ambulance company so I knew the head of the hospital's emergency services very well. I called and asked him if this guy was ok. He informed me that he was off the drugs, only takes a nip now and then, and most of his malpractice suits have been settled. I hung up the phone and told him he would do and was highly recommended. Unfortunately, I could not have the procedure done for at least a week. I left the hospital with a case of nitroglycerin and made it through the week..

Cheryl brought me to the hospital and made sure I had everything I needed to get through the night. Hand held video games, magazines and a book I was reading. The next thing I knew it, was morning and I was getting ready for surgery. From this point until I awoke in the recovery room, I have no clue what happened.

I woke up in the recovery room and my parents and Cheryl were there. My kids Shauna and Jeff from a previous marriage are too little or too small to be allowed in. I had to wait to see them, and that bothered me because I knew they needed to see me to make sure I was all right. My parents, left and my wife stayed with me. I hated having the ET tube still in my mouth—it was so dry my wife had to keep passing ice cubes across my lips. It was at this time that the surgeon informed me that while they had my chest open he determined it prudent to perform two additional grafts. So I had a quintuple bypass. Believe it or not, there is something good that happened; I have no heart damage at all. This really made me feel great. My stepdaughter Tiffany was going to stay at home while Cheryl stayed with me. About eight o'clock, Cheryl got a call about a murder in the building next to ours. She needed to leave to stay with Tiff. This was not a problem, except that evening around midnight or so, I went into respiratory arrest. This is a very important tip, if you have sleep apnea please tell your doctor.

Sleep apnea and morphine do not mix well at all. Throughout the whole arrest I knew what was going as well as seeing what was going on. This really astounded the staff that brought me back. As a matter of fact, latter in the week one of the doctors asked me if I was looking down at what was going on; I told him no, that I was looking up. After I thought about it, this is not a good sign. Anyway, they got me back and low and behold here comes the Endo Tracheal tube again.

The next day, everyone was standing around my bed whispering. I motioned to the nurse to get me a pen and paper. She handed it to me and I wrote, "I know." Everyone was shocked that I knew what happened but naturally relieved I was ok. It was about this time that something strange occurred. As I was reflecting on what happened I felt this sense of serenity and completeness pass over me, it felt as though that if I didn't make it everything would be all right. I had no fear or did not feel nervous about anything that happened so far. I was supposed to go home after four days, but they enrolled me into sleep school, which I could not go to until my eighth day. This was by far the dumbest thing they had me do. The days following my surgery I could not sleep. I do not believe I got more that 3 hours sleep in 5 days. So the sleep test was not very successful. I would be going home with a breathing machine. This whole time I was in the hospital, except for the night before and the night of my surgery, Cheryl was with me the whole time. She slept in the bed while I slept in the cardiac chair. This meant a lot to me and I think it helped with my recovery having someone so dedicated by my side. My first wife, Sheila, brought the kids each day to visit me. This also meant a lot, she did not have to do this. I am probably the only man that can say he ended up with not one but two terrific ex-wives. I probably should have mentioned that my doctor categorized my personality. We have type A, type B, etc. Well, I a.m. type A+. He thought about my going to a stress reduction class but determined that it would not be fair to the Instructor. He thought I might stress him out. When I went for my first office visit after my surgery, the doctor was twenty five minutes late, he proceeded to knock on the door and asked me if it was safe to come in. I had to laugh, because after my hospital stay, I decided that I was not going to let things bother me, and I would think things through before I reacted. This has worked somewhat okay over the last four years. Still, can get a little riled though. Because of the amount of time I spent in the cardiac chair, my shoulders were very sore and I was in a lot of pain. I could only do lower bodywork at cardiac rehab and had to go to physical therapy for my shoulders. I did not last long at cardiac rehab, because the nurse and I got in a major disagreement and I decided to work out at the gym. That's another story.

I am 45 now, and it has been a little over four years since my surgery. Except for not being able to stick to a diet or eat the right foods, I am doing and feeling all right. My daughter has high cholesterol and my son borderline, and I hope they do not have to go through what I have been through. As I reflect on what happened to me during this critical time, I am convinced that someone was watching over me. I am not the most religious person, but I believe I was taken care of for a purpose. I do not know what the purpose is yet, but when it happens I will know.

Jay Sylvain

*Heart valve replacement surgery can be necessary when a valve becomes diseased, and does not operate smoothly. The heart's valves are responsible for keeping the blood flowing in a one-way direction within the heart. When a valve becomes diseased, they may fail to open and close freely, which can disrupt the normal flow of blood within the heart. Modern medicine has successfully mastered valve replacement, and that gives many patients a new lease on life. Susan shares her new valve replacement with you in order to help alleviate some of the fears that you may experience if you face this type of surgery.*

*"Guard the good deposit that was entrusted to you, guard it with the help of the Holy Spirit who lives in us."*
*2 Timothy 1:14*

# Heart Value Replacement
## By
## Susan Rosier

11 Dec 1999

I am 41 years old, and in a month it will be a year since my Heart Valve Replacement surgery. Here is my story:I was born with a heart problem but I didn't know exactly what it was until I was in my early twenties. When I was little, they said it could have been a multitude of things, but not to worry; just live a normal life. So I did. I had just moved into a new house and was feeling a little extra tired, so I decided it was time to have my heart checked, as I did periodically while growing up. The doctor decided to do a heart catherization and the news was a bit surprising. He stressed to me as he explained the results that it was important that I knew and understood what the problem was.

I had aortic valve deficiency with mild stenosis. It sounded scary to me and was a lot more to be concerned about than I ever thought.

He told me I was young and healthy, and if I took care of myself and took my antibiotics when I went to the dentist and tried to avoid infections, that I could probably go for another 50 years and by then it would be a piece of cake.

I made it until I was 38 and pregnant with my son. I went for my yearly check-up that was always the same. My valve seemed loud to me though. The doctor would always mention how loud it was. I could hear it at night in bed.

Well, my readings started to change, and I was really having a tough time with this pregnancy. Plus, I had a five-year old at home. My cardiologist suggested that I not go into labor and to have him two weeks early by C-section. My first child was 10 lb. 3 oz. and he didn't want to chance me going into labor with another big one. He was born and things were fine. He was 8 lb. 4 oz.

The cardiologist said to come back in three months and get another ultra sound. I did and he said everything looks like it was good and my readings are back where they used to be. Well, I was having trouble breathing and coughing and heartburn terribly. He said it was most likely reflux brought on by pregnancy and told me to take Pepcid. I did just that, but I sure had a hard time. I even went to a pulmonary doctor and a gastro doctor and they all said reflux. I was on reflux medication for a year. It helped some but I started to have spasms in my chest. It was like when you go outside and breathe really cold air or drink cold water—Oh, how your chest hurts! It happens a lot, even walking or anything. I carried my son from our condo to the beach about two blocks and by the time I got to the water I was doubled over rubbing my chest. I would say, "Boy, what did I eat to do this." It went on for six months and it was time for another check up from the cardiologist.

I was having a sonagram done and the technician said, "Wow, do you have any trouble with this valve?" "Did you ever consider getting a new one?" Hummmm, Why did he ask that? Well, in the doctor's office, I was telling him about these spasms and he looked at me as if he had heard me for the first time. He said, "You need a heart catherization soon." So a week later, there I was and then I was told that the valve was calcified to the point that the blood was having a hard time getting through the tiny hole, and that was why the spasms and pain. It was time to replace the valve and soon.

One month later, I had the surgery. I still don't know how I got there that morning, I was in a state for sure. I had two small children and I was gonna be down for three months and maybe more. That's enough to blow a mother's mind. But I had to do it to be here for them for longer than I was headed for. Thank God for modern medicine. I had a St. Jude's mechanical valve placed where my old worn aortic valve was. Here I am in good shape to chase that two-year-old boy. It's wonderful.

One thing I would like to hit on, and that is the emotional side of this surgery. I had heard some people suffer depression, but not all. The surgeon told me that for some reason, his younger patients have much more pain, also. Well, I figured I am pretty upbeat and this was gonna be the surgery to cure all. Why would I be depressed? I can tell you I ran a close second to the wicked witch on the Wizard of Oz. I laid a few nurses out and cried and cried a river the first couple of weeks after my surgery. My emotions were so crazy and anytime someone did something nice for my family and I, the water works would roll. My husband hated to see the flower truck come around the corner because he knew it would trigger it. The pain and helplessness were terrible after I came home. I was in the hospital a week and still couldn't tend to my personal needs when I got home. Fortunately, I have a wonderful husband. He sure got a workout between the kids and I. The trouble is now, I owe him big.

My mother was a wonderful help, too and boy, did I need them. The pain was very bad in my chest, and I had a stabbing pain under my breast for the first month that took my breath away. I realized I had acid reflux on top of all this and had to cough more then the average person.

Boy, that was a challenge. I had a heart pillow almost flat from squeezing it. Geez! All that ever could hurt did for a long time, and the depression got worse and worse. I was not getting well fast enough. I got a terrible cold right away, and for three weeks I was weak and so dizzy I could not see straight. I found out my iron was very low and that I had a low thyroid. So I started my medications for that and a lot of vitamins to start building up myself again. Still, after six months, I was in tears at about six in the evening and moody all the time. I was very impatient with my children. I hated the way I was. I never thought anything was funny and my husband must have gotten sick of my tears and gripes of coping with the days, but he never said a word. He just looked worn out. I really looked at him and saw the wear on him one day, I thought I need to do something. I called my doctor and asked for a mild antidepressant to try. He started me out on a low dose and in two weeks I could see a difference. In a month I saw a huge difference. I took my hubby away for a weekend and we laughed and enjoyed it so much, I wish they would have suggested much sooner that I take something for a while to help with all the anxiety I had suffered.

My doctor knows me very well, and I feel as though he should have saved me sooner from this. I haven't cried in so long and my energy level is better. My household is much happier because Mom is her old self. This is something I want to stress to women and men my age, or ones with a lot of responsibilities on their shoulders. This surgery takes it away from you for awhile and if you are like me, you want to be super person and break all the records for recovery. It would only set me back more. I think I was susceptible to more colds and everything because I was stressed, and I kept getting knocked down. I believe in my new fixed heart, that an antidepressant should be offered along with this surgery. I am headed for a hysterectomy the month after my one-year anniversary to heart surgery and I am a bit gun shy, but I feel as though I made it through a "biggy" last year, so this is gonna be a piece of cake.

Only we, who have been there, can possibly understand what heart surgery is all about. I wake up everyday and am so grateful to be here, to hear that welcome ticking in my chest, and to be able to see those two sweet angels in my house looking up to me.

Susan Rosier

*Tony's experience is beautifully expressed from the heart of a spiritual man. His faith and surrender to place himself into God's hands speak for itself as a testimony of God's grace and love.*

*"Let us then approach the throne of grace with confidence, so that we may receive mercy and find grace to help us in our hour of need."*
*Hebrews 4:16*

# In God's Hands
## By
## Tony Purcell

At the age of 45, and with no prior major health problems, I went to my doctor complaining of abdominal discomfort. After a couple months treatment for what was thought to be an intestinal disorder, I took a turn for the worse and was admitted into emergency for congestive heart failure. After a day of tests, my doctor came in and informed my wife and myself that my diagnosis was cardiomyopathy and I would probably need a new heart within a year.

In the blink of an eye, I went from a relatively active life, capable of arduous work, to hiking in the mountains, and an occasional day of surfing with my sons, to lying in a hospital bed witnessing the ebbing of my physical existence. Granted, many people get less than a blink of an eye, but for some we get to contemplate our situation and find either positive or negative ways of dealing with it.

At first I experienced mostly shock, as I had no expectation of this diagnosis or any knowledge of heart transplantation being more than an experimental remedy. After this, I had various periods of denial, "Why me?" depression, loneliness, even terror at my situation. Throughout this period of negativity, God reminded me, of His presence through the prayers and cards of many of my friends and relatives. His showed me in His holy word, the Bible, assurance that He was in control and that I needn't fear death.

He also showed how He could work through doctors and latest scientific discoveries. With a variety of medications, I was able to return to all my former activities with relative normalcy. I acknowledged God's hand in my recovery but to be honest, attributed most of His works coming through medical science and the will of my body to survive. I found later that God planned to teach me more of His power and grace and the importance of putting all my trust and faith in Him.

My medicated fix was to be only temporary, and after three years my condition worsened. In mid-November of 1994, I was put on the waiting list for a donor heart. While on the waiting list and tethered to a beeper, I was still somewhat functional both at work and at home, so I still had my moments of denial to the seriousness of my health. Things started to become more real when on New Years' Eve, as my family and I were exiting our home to go to a community celebration, the phone rang. It was the hospital calling to say a heart was available and to come in for surgery.

I remember the drive quite well. I felt some sense of irony as to my driving to get a transplant but it helped to keep my mind off my worry to concentrate on getting us there safely on New Years' Eve. I remember thinking how this might be the last time I would be with my family. It made my eyes swell up with tears when I thought how I might not be around to see my son graduate from high school and from college. I thought how I would miss seeing the success of my older son and how I might not be here to help stand by him in his failures. I thought how I would miss my wife's courage and support, and her insistence that everything would turn out all right and be to God's glory.

Well, we made it to the hospital in an hour and I was prepared for surgery. On the way the phone rang. After hanging up, the nurse informed me that surgery had been cancelled when it was found that the donor heart was not suitable for transplanting. This occurs sometimes because the heart is the last organ to be harvested from a donor, and occasionally a defect or some other reason is found to make it unsuitable. Needless to say, this roller coaster ride was distressful and disheartening.

Approximately two weeks later, my condition worsened and I was put into intensive care (not a very fun place to be). At this point any denial I had was fading fast. I would stand next to my bed and do knee bends and other stretching exercises to try to keep my muscles from atrophying. I felt I needed to try to do something to keep my body in as good a shape as I could in order to survive my transplant, if and when it occurred. I still had some idea that there might be something I could do to increase my chances for survival.

I did take great comfort in reading my Bible and in the passages that God led me to. Also comforting were the prayers of many friends and relatives, and visits from family and church family, when they were allowed in. Still, with all that was going on with me physically, many times I was more into my illness than into God, and counted on others to intervene in my behalf.

On February 3, my wife's birthday, I was informed that a donor heart was available and off I went by ambulance to the transplant hospital. It makes for a good story now, but at the time finding out that this heart was also not suitable for transplanting was starting to try my faith.

Coming back to intensive care, I was finally coming to terms with my incarceration. There were going to be only two ways out of this situation (transplant or death), and considering the physical and mental ordeal I was experiencing, going home to my maker was starting to get a larger percentage of my vote.

On February 13, a friend visited me for a while. Before leaving he prayed for me. After he left, I began to get really depressed. While lying there all "tubed-up," monitors beeping, and being aware of others in the ward in even worse conditions than myself, I was greatly overwhelmed by my situation. I felt totally helpless, scared, and alone. It was at that time that that I cried out unto my Lord (as David had many times in Psalms) to deliver me out of my helplessness and distress. For the first time in this ordeal I totally gave my condition to God. I acknowledged my own helplessness and the inability of anyone else to save me. After my prayer, I truly knew that it was all in God's hands and that His will would be done. Whatever, that will was, I was prepared to accept it and to praise it. Peace and contentment was upon me and at approximately 11 p.m. I drifted off to sleep.

An hour and twenty minutes later at 12: 20 a.m., February 14, 1995, a nurse came and woke me up with the news that "We have a heart for you." This time it was a keeper. Surgery took about two hours, and a week later I was able to walk out of the hospital. God had given me two Valentine's Day gifts. One was a new heart for me and the other was a new heart for God.

I am soon going to celebrate my fifth year anniversary. I'm working full time, getting a mountain bicycle for Christmas, (don't tell my wife I peeked) and have had many memorable times surfing with my sons. God has indeed blessed me, and I give Praise to Jesus. Believe it or not, I still have times when I think situations have to be resolved through my effort's, that if you worry about something long enough that the solution will finally come to you. But deep down in my heart I know that it's all in God's hands.

Tony Purcell

*Coronary heart disease is in a large part due to the interaction of genetic traits with environmental issues such as diet, exercise, smoking, body fat and other factors. Genetic traits that contribute to heart disease risk can be identified in approximately 80% of heart disease patients. First-degree relatives, brother/sister, sons/daughters can have the same genetic trait. Possible preventive cardiology can be achieved by carefully screening such family members and provide valuable data for genetic research.*

*"If you believe, you will receive whatever you ask for in prayer."*
*Matthew 21:22*

# Myocardial Infarction with Stent Placement

Hi, my name is Jeri.

I am 40 years old, and I had a heart attack two weeks after my 40th birthday. I am female, and married with four kids.

I guess I kind of knew by some intuition that I was going to have a heart attack, because both of my parents have heart disease. My father had bypass in his late 40's and my mom had two heart attacks with the first one in her early 50's. I had chest pain on and off for quite a while. I even remember an event during PE in middle school.

After going to the hospital by ambulance and given and EKG, they said it was a heart attack and I was given TPA, put in ICU for 3 days and then transferred to another hospital. I was given a cardiac catherization and they inserted a stent. I recovered with no apparent damage to my heart. (woo-hoo) It's been a month now and in a few days I am going to have a thallium stress test. I would do anything not to go through another cardiac catherization again. It was horrible.

Emotionally, I feel like I will never be the same. I cry every day, at least once a day. I feel better physically than I do mentally. I feel 90 years old and I hope I will not feel this way forever. Oh, forgot, I did smoke a pack a day, had high cholesterol and a family history. So I guess I had three strikes against me. So at this point, I'm really scared still and very depressed.

Jeri

*Jeri was so kind to write her mother's heart story for the book. As you can see the family genetics appear to play a major role. Thank you, Jeri, for sharing your mom's story with us.*

*"Look to the Lord and his strength; seek his face always."*
*1 Chronicles 16:11*

# Myocardial Infarction
## by
## Jeri's Mom

They had just moved to a rural town in Nevada when my mom had bad pain in her upper back. She had already had a heart attack four years earlier and had angioplasty. This time, she knew it was her heart and they went to the only hospital in town. A physician's assistant saw her. After evaluating her, the physician's assistant told her she hurt her back from moving and gave her pain medication and sent her home. A few hours later she was back in a full-blown heart attack. After having an EKG, which was simultaneously sent to a large hospital in Reno, and her blood drawn, the cardiologist in Reno told the doctor treating her (who was an osteopath) to give her TPA. Well, he would not, because he said he did not feel comfortable giving her TPA. He felt she was not having a heart attack. She was to be airlifted to Reno, but because of high winds, she had to be taken in an ambulance. With her was the local cable installer, who volunteers as an EMT, by her side. He could not give her any medication—not an aspirin if she needed it. Finally, in Reno she was given TPA and angioplasted. She was placed on a machine to make her heart work minimally and this caused kidney failure. As a result, she has tremendous damage to her heart. I'm sure there are a million little details I don't know, but this is the gist of it.

She is alive, her life is definitely not the same, and she is suing the doctor who refused the TPA.

Thank you,

Jeri

*Carol, as a young single mom, relates her experience with the fear of not knowing combined with the fear of having a small child totally dependent on her. Her spiritual faith guided her way as carefully as if she were carried, as in the story "footprints in the sand."*

*"I will lie down and sleep in peace, for you alone, O Lord make me dwell in safety."*
*Psalm 4:8*

# Sinus Node Virus
## By
## Carol Adams

Hope this helps:

I am a 39 year old female, my occupation is a nurse (LPN) and I work 11-7 shift at night at the local nursing home. I also have one child, age 5. My experience, now that I look back, it started about six months ago. Then I was having some weakness, low stamina, and edema in my lower legs and hands, along with palpitations. But they began as very subtle signs, hardly noticeable. On September 10, 1999, I was up in the Kiamanchi Mountains on a women's retreat. I was taking Lasix, 40 mg twice a day, and Potassium at the time for edema. I had about a nine to ten pound weight loss in 2 days from that alone. I was staying overnight there. I noticed a little difficulty breathing and I got tired easily. I would get short of breath just from climbing stairs. We also had a small hill to climb. I couldn't do it without stopping to catch my breath. I took it pretty easy the rest of the weekend; I was on vacation anyway. It wasn't really bad enough to get my attention. Even before this I as having little episodes of my heart palpating or feeling as it was going to run away, but only lasting a few seconds.

On September 15, I had a really bad spell of my heart racing and I felt like I was going to pass out. I was at McDonald's and it was approximately 12 noon. I am not diabetic but I felt like my blood sugar was low. It had been since 2 a.m. since I had eaten. I tried to eat some French fries, but it made me feel worse. At this time, I was getting a little concerned. It had be approximately 30-45 minutes with no relief. I felt weak, nauseated, cold and clammy, and felt as though my chest was going to explode.

My daughter had an appointment at the rehabilitation center across town. I drove out there, but still wasn't feeling any better. The therapist who came to get my daughter to take her for therapy asked me if I was doing okay. I am one that doesn't ask for help, but I was a little scared by now. It had been a little over an hour since the episode started. The therapist went to get a nurse; they checked my blood sugar it was 109 (normal). They checked my blood pressure 90/44, which is quite low for me. Pulse was 44 (normal 60-88) per minute. Never had any heart trouble before. This scared me even more. The staff there put me in a bed and ran an EKG. It showed bradycardia with premature ventricular contractions and premature atrial contractions with several in a row. They called my sister in town and had her take me to the hospital. I was admitted for observation and tests.

I had several blood tests, and they all came back normal. All the tests, thallium scan and drug induced stress test and echocardiogram came back normal. I had a consult with a cardiologist on September 21, 1999. He couldn't find anything either. But why was I having syncope episodes? Something was wrong. They put me on an event recorder to catch some of the episodes. I was thankful for the primary care physician that wouldn't give up. The primary care physician knew what was wrong (Sick Sinus Syndrome) but could not get the cardiologist to agree.

I went back to work for 2 days and I couldn't even do a bed check without stopping. On September 27, 1999, I had another bad episode, only this time it went the other way. Pulse >160. The whole time from

September 15th, 1999, I was running a pulse rate of approximately 35-50 beats per minute. This time, I was able to catch it on the event monitor and send it in. I was taken to the emergency room and admitted for observation. I was discharged the next day.

Another consult was made to an electrophysiologist in Tulsa, Oklahoma on October 1, 1999. I went to this office; they had tried to cancel but missed us. He was called out on an emergency. At that point, I was desperate to find out what the problem was. I demanded that we stay until we could see him. We met him a 5 p.m. An appointment was set for a cardiac catherization (Electrophysiology Study) on Monday October 4, 1999. I went to Tulsa for the catherization. I got there and it was cancelled because of the doctor being sick. It was finally rescheduled for Monday, October 4, 1999. This was pretty scary. My dad had one and couldn't remember it. There again, it doesn't pay to have knowledge about a procedure. Especially to know the things that can go wrong, and the dangers of the procedure. Sometimes you can have too much knowledge.

I was then told that I had had a virus that damaged the sinus node of the heart, and I would probably in two to three months have to have a pacemaker put in. The doctor started me on medication to slow the atrial fibrillation down to prevent the syncope episodes, but it also slowed the heart rate down. Now my pulse rate was running in the 30-40's.

I was still wearing the event monitor, and feeling worse on October 14, 1999. I was recording about every 45 minutes to 1 hour and sending it in. The monitoring place called me back and wanted me to keep monitoring. I knew I wasn't feeling really good. This was about 12p.m. When I called the doctor's office to tell them I was on my way, my rate was below 20 per minute. I was able to keep alert and sent someone to take me to the doctor's office. Then they transferred me to Tulsa, to a major hospital. When I arrived there, they inserted a pacemaker the next morning on October 14, 1999.

I look back now and realize just how God watched over me and took care of me. I am a single mom and could have really been in a lot of trouble, but He was able to keep me alert enough to get help. There was no one with me at the time. The peace that I felt during this time of illness was awesome. I give God the credit for my recovery (which was approximately two months time). God isn't finished with me yet! I still have a 5-year-old daughter to raise. She is another very special gift from God. The emotional side of this was very hard. Especially during all the ups and downs of not knowing what was wrong and knowing what could happen. I had many questions in my mind. Will I be able to go back to work? There was that possibility mentioned by the doctors. Will I ever get my strength up? How was I going to provide a living? If it wasn't for the support of my family and the prayers of my church family, I don't think I would have made it except for the reassurance of the doctors and nurses who happen to be very close friends. Probably the hardest thing I had to do was to ask for help, (I am very independent) and to be a patient. You see, I am usually taking care of patients with this kind of problem.

Thanks,

Carol Adams

*"God is our refuge and strength, an ever-present help in trouble."*
*Psalm 46:1*

# Coronary Artery Disease—Hypertensive Heart Disease
## By
## Candy Stowe

29 December 1999

On July 29, 1999, I woke to my alarm as usual. I felt exhausted. But I got up anyway, as this was my only day off this week. I fixed my coffee and sat down to wake up. I decided to take my laundry down the hall to the washer to get that going. The only other thing I planned on doing was grocery shopping. As I walked back to the kitchen I was dizzy and very tired. I decided to check my blood pressure—194/114. I rechecked it. It remained the same. I had not checked my blood pressure since the last of June when I stayed home from work for three days not feeling well. I had been under a lot of pressure at work from personnel issues and management matters for months. I decided to go back to bed and sleep a little more. Maybe I would feel better. I had already slept fourteen hours. I woke up again three hours later. My son came to visit, my daughter called, and I went shopping. I was ready for sleep again by 11 p.m.

I awoke the next day to the alarm. Still tired, I called in to my job. I told my boss my blood pressure was elevated. He urged me to go to the doctor.

I went to the emergency room on July 30. I was told to see a doctor for follow-up and needed a stress test. On August 3, I went to a doctor who increased my blood pressure medicine, again said I needed a stress test. My blood pressure was 202/110. A week later, I returned to the same clinic. My blood pressure was still elevated; I felt like I had a bad flu. I was again told I needed a stress test. I finally understood I needed to see a cardiologist and made an appointment for the following week. On August 17, I started the stress test at the cardiologist's office. I tired quickly on the treadmill and asked if it was going too fast. He lowered the speed, but I took two more steps and fainted. I awoke briefly at the bottom of the treadmill to hear the doctor say no one had ever fainted before and my EKG did not even change. My next memory is being lifted to a sitting position. The doctor was sitting in front of me. I could only see where I was looking no side vision or awareness of anything else going on. I wasn't scared, but I was aware that I could feel nothing, no pain or sensations and my thinking was impaired.

Two days later, I had the dobutamine stress test and in less than a minute coded. The doctor brought me back, but at the end of the test I was not able to think. I was mostly asleep for a total of five weeks. I was awake for about five hours a day. My blood pressure was brought under control. I slowly have regained partially my strength. I have had 3 months of cardiac rehabilitation and a.m. starting physical therapy for one month. It is now Dec. 1999 and I am trying to go back to work two days a week.

I hope you like my story.
Candy R. Stowe

*Here is the story of a mother's courage to fight the day to day battles with a child's illness. God's grace is sufficient and he will not forsake his little ones.*

*"The Lord is my shepherd, I shall not want."*
*Psalm 23:1*

# A Child's Struggle With Congenital Heart Disease
## Told by his Mother
## Mathew's Story

When Mathew was born, his father was in the Marine Corps stationed in California. At his six-week checkup, his pediatrician found a heart murmur. They believed he had a hole in his heart and referred him to Balboa Naval Hospital in San Diego. He was put on medication to help control his symptoms, but by the time he was 4 months old he was suffering from heart failure. They did a heart catherization and found that he had a Patent Ductus Arteriosis. The Ductus Arteriosis is an artery that bypasses the blood to the lungs before birth. It is supposed to close on it's own when the baby is born and starts using the lungs. They told us it would be a relatively easy operation to tie off this artery and Mathew would be perfectly normal. What a relief this was, after thinking he had a hole in his heart!

But after the surgery, instead of getting better, Mathew became worse. Two and a half weeks went by until the doctors finally decided to do another heart catherization to find out why he was deteriorating. They found the PDA was still open. Mathew was then sent to the University of San Diego where they performed immediate surgery and found that the Naval Hospital had tied off his left pulmonary artery instead of the PDA. They closed the PDA and tried to save his left pulmonary artery but were unsuccessful. The use of Mathew's left lung was gone forever. Mathew's father left the Marine Corp as soon as his release date came and we moved back to Iowa. In the mean time, Mathew developed a leaky Mitral Valve. When he was 21 months old, he received an artificial Mitral Valve at the University of Iowa. He did very well with this valve for many years. In the summer of 1996 it was decided that he had outgrown this valve and needed a larger one. It is very hard to replace a small valve with a larger valve but the surgery went very well. But Mathew didn't improve. Instead he developed an atrial automatic tachycardia (abnormal heartbeat) which is being controlled by medicine. He is also suffering from chronic pulmonary hypertension, which is mainly caused from the lost left pulmonary artery and he has developed another leaky valve. He is very under-weight and small for his age and has little interest in eating so now he will be hooked up at night to a pump that will feed him. Fortunately, this will be done at home. We have come to the point where the doctors aren't sure what the next step is, but we take one day at a time and know with much prayer Mathew will get through this too.

*Helen Holshouer has written her heart disease experience for us in detail in order that the procedure she under went could be fully understood. It is one of the latest surgeries developed to help to restore blood flow to diseased coronary vessels. Her emotional and physical experience is dramatic, but Helen shares with you her courage in coping with this experience. In reading her accounts, scripture reminds me of the magnificence of God's hand in our lives.*

*"Now to him who is able to do immeasurably more than all we ask or imagine, according to his power that is at work in us."*
*Ephesians 3: 20*

# My Lifesaving Heart Surgery
By
Helen Y. Holshouser
Transmyocardial Revascularization (TMR)


April, 19, 1999

This was a Monday, the day that I got the first inclination that I had heart disease, but I was in total denial! I am a 50 year old woman married to Max for 28 years now, with two daughters; Ali a college student, and Annie a senior in high school. Professionally, I am a master's level psychologist, working in public mental health, providing individual, child, marriage, and group therapy. I worked long hours, because I felt "called" to be a counselor. In the last year or so, I'd started a new program for men that battered, a group of people I never expected to counsel, but work I found challenging and rewarding. As I look back, I had been getting sicker and sicker over a year, maybe several years, but especially those last six months. After working long hours I often felt I hardly had the energy to drive home. More and more often, my husband cooked dinner, and I slept most of the weekend, feeling "sick." I went to a family doctor regularly, at least once a month. She attributed my lack of energy to stress, my anemia, and diabetes. It made sense to me. In January 1999, I'd had a scare, thinking I might have ovarian or uterine cancer. But a biopsy in February proved benign cysts. I was stressed to be sure. My mother had had her first heart attack at age 50, and I was now that very age, but I mentioned that possibility to my doctor, and her partner even did an EKG sometime during that fall of 1998. Apparently it was normal, and he was not concerned. Twice in the week before this date, I experienced "spells" of feeling sick enough that I called my husband to come pick me up, feeling dizzy, faint, sweaty, short of breath. Once I had taken the car in for repairs and had walked across the street to wait in a café. By the time I got there, a two-block walk, I was sick. I assumed I was having a low blood sugar problem, and wrote a note to the restaurant clerk who promptly called my husband to come and get me. After having something to eat and resting, I felt okay—I didn't even test my blood sugar! Then last night, April 18th, after feeling sick and worn out all weekend, I'd gone to the grocery store for the family's weekly trip. As I rounded each aisle, I felt worse, shakier, short of breath, disoriented. I tried to kind of hurry, thinking I'd cut the trip short and go on home. By the time I reached the check out lanes however, I knew I was too sick to drive home. I actually thought I was going to faint trying to stand there and check out. I started to ask the clerk to call Max, but I was embarrassed to do that again. So I half stumbled to the pay phone, and could hardly function as I searched for change. I couldn't think straight; what change did I need? What was my phone number? I got Max, who could get there in 5 minutes! I was trying to put on a brave front, but I was tearful as I asked a bag boy to please put the groceries in my car. I had no chest pain, and I truly thought it was low blood sugar, which I had dealt with before, so I wasn't too worried about sitting in the dark car, in a dark parking lot until my husband arrived to take me home. I started to cry as my husband arrived and comforted me. As I waited for him to arrive, I assured the bag boy that I was all right. It did occur to me that this seemed worse than it had in a long time, and maybe I was stupid to have come out to sit in the car alone and wait. What if I died out here, no one would know? Then I felt stupid for feeling that way, and in minutes Max pulled up and I felt safe. This time, when I got home I actually tested my blood sugar, it was not low, it was normal. I was surprised. I lay on the couch, feeling too weak to move practically; wondering what in the world could cause such a thing, other than my blood sugar. I did wonder about my heart, but dismissed that as not likely. This time it took me lying on the couch for about two hours before I felt some energy returning. I got up gingerly, packed lunches for the next day, and went to bed. The next morning, I awakened feeling much better, greeted my 16 year old, and said goodbye to my husband as he left early for work. I showered and dressed myself for work. I think I even fed the cat and dog, and made breakfast for my daughter, and myself. I seemed fine until minutes before we were headed out the door, when suddenly I felt faint, and had no choice but to lie down or I felt, fall down! I was shocked, but the feeling passed quickly, and in 10 minutes, I was ready to leave the house taking my child to school on the way to work. In all honesty, I was worried, but I was unsure what to do. As luck would have it, I had had a falling out with my family doctor, and had decided to change to an internist in my own small town. My first appointment with him was coming up this Thursday, in 4 days. So I was "between doctors," and unsure what to do. I thought I would ask the nurses at work for some advice. I wondered if it was a problem with my heart, if a doctor could even tell today, what had happened last night. Of course, this Monday was a day that would not stop, filled with emergency needs of others. It was around 4p.m. I believe, before I got around to talking to the nurses. I was surprised to find myself tearing up as I recalled the night before and the morning's events. My friends urged me in no uncertain terms to seek medical attention right away. Still, I kept hemming and hawing, thinking maybe, I should wait until Thursday when, I would see my new doctor. But I had to admit, I hadn't felt well all day, and as I drove home I felt increasingly bad, so I decided to stop at the urgent care center newly opened in our town. I couldn't believe that I felt out of breath walking 20 feet across the floor, and felt I would faint while I tried to sign in! I was probably very lucky that a former emergency room doctor was there that night. He listened to me and ordered an EKG. I'm still unsure what he saw there, because he was very calm and reassuring to me as he said he thought I was okay. He called the hospital and wanted me to go directly there "just for a couple of tests." I was shocked when he then wanted to send me by ambulance! I had worked all day, driven myself there, and lived five minutes away. He finally, gave in to my pleading to let my husband transport me. He gave me nitroglycerin to take with me if I had chest pains; I had none. I truly thought I was going to meet a doctor at the hospital to do a stress test, and as it was about 7 p.m. then, I expected to be home by 9 p.m.. When I called my husband I wasn't even particularly upset, and didn't think my teenager should go with us, but should stay home and do homework. When we walked into our local hospital, they were waiting for us. They had me in an alcove in the emergency room immediately, wiring me up to all kinds of things! It seemed they thought I was an emergency, and I kept saying "you're making a mistake, I just came for some tests, I'm supposed to meet a doctor for a couple tests and then go home." I actually made them check their charts, and they returned saying yes, we have the right person, we think you might be having a heart attack! I said my first "You're kidding!" of what must have been fifty "You're kidding" that night! They did several tests, I don't even know what all, and finally told us about 11 p.m. or so that "I think that you need to stay overnight." "You're kidding!" I said. (Denial is an incredible thing!) The next day there were more tests, including I think, a treadmill stress test which I obviously failed because within a minute I was passing out! The doctors kept saying to wait, they'd give us information by lunchtime, or supper time, or 8 p.m. and we'd probably get to go home then. Then at 9 p.m., they said I needed to stay for more tests the next day, They need to do nuclear scans, and they called in a cardiologist. I also was relieved that the new internist, I had planned to start with on Thursday was notified by the urgent care doctor, and he claimed me, so I didn't feel that I was without a doctor. Of course, we didn't know each other, and I was scared and sick and unsure, but he was very kind to take me on. I think it was Tuesday or Wednesday night when I met the cardiologist who informed me that they would do a catherization the next day, or maybe Friday. But maybe I'd go home and come back as an outpatient and do it. She actually said, that she doubted that I had a major heart problem, and that she thought it was probably a blood pressure problem. I was relieved to hear that! Then she said that if the catherization did show blockages, she would recommend that they proceed immediately with an angioplasty. My internist had already talked about my possible need for bypass, telling me that angioplasties don't tend to last well in diabetics. I was so confused! I think I had the catherization on Thursday. Immediately afterwards, the cardiologist told my husband and me, (but I was groggy) and our minister that had waited with my husband, that I had many diffuse blockages and that they could not do angioplasties or bypass on me. They had decided to treat me medically. As I became more alert, I tried to ask her several times to explain things to me exactly. She said, on several occasions, "Just wait until you come to see me in my office where I will have your report in front of me and a model of the heart, and I will explain it to you completely." I was surprised then to learn that I wasn't scheduled to see her for a month! Then her office called and actually put off my appointment with her for two more weeks. That meant I was being sent home from the hospital on a bunch of new medications, knowing I now have coronary heart disease, but I did not have a heart attack. I had an appointment with the cardiologist in six weeks! It appeared that my new internist would really be treating the heart disease, as he wrote the prescriptions and I had a return appointment to see him within the week. I went home thinking, okay, I'm lucky, I have heart disease, but it must not be too bad, I didn't have a heart attack, they didn't have to operate, I'll take these medications and be back at work next week probably. Little did I know or understand what lay ahead for me.

After spending that first momentous week in the local hospital, I was sent home with a bunch of new medicines, to regulate my heartbeat, and I'm not sure what else. I was assigned to start cardiac rehabilitation in a couple weeks, and thought I'd go back at work by then or soon after. Having arrived home on April 23, 1999, this is an e-mail I wrote to a friend at work on May 6, 1999.

Dear Katherine,

Surprise! Get this I have learned to e-mail! I'm happy to report that I am feeling better and to actually be sitting up at the computer. What a shock the way this knocked me off my feet! Thanks so much for the note and the doctor names. I may use them yet, but for now I'm waiting to start cardiac rehab tomorrow and see what advice I get. My internist did tell me last week that if I had to have surgery, they would send me to the University Hospital, which made me feel better on first wash, then worried me as he explained that they didn't have the means to do the surgery here. Tonight, I saw that he wrote that I had "inoperable coronary artery disease" on my family leave application! That set me back! I guess I hadn't quite understood that they couldn't operate, more that they weren't choosing to at this time, or that it wasn't necessary. However, Dean Ornish says heart disease can be reversed. I have to make the major changes required. I'm already realizing keeping my determination will be difficult—incredible when you consider the alternative—we'll see.

I really didn't mean to go on. Give everyone my love and tell them that I hope to return next week at least part time.

See you then,

Helen

Friday, May 7th, I did start a cardiac rehabilitation program. If was close to my place of work, which I thought, would be helpful when I returned to work soon. Sunday May 9th, was Mother's Day. I was happy that my college daughter could come home, and was looking forward to spending the day with the family. Actually, I hated to tell them, but I wasn't feeling very well, having some angina, but I didn't need to do much anyway so I tried to just be loving and gracious. The girls had planned to purchase some flowers for me and plant them in the garden in front of the house, which I usually did this time of year. It was obvious I unable to do this year. I had told them that would be my favorite gift from them. It was very hot however, and I just didn't feel like going out early in the day. We waited until 4 or 5p.m. hoping it would be cooler. I thought it wouldn't hurt to just ride in the car with them to help choose the flowers. I didn't plan to get out, or walk around in the heat much. We got to the first garden center, and I tried to get out just to look a little. I had immediate angina and dizziness, so I got back in the air-conditioned car and pointed to specimens, I thought look good and those precious girls brought them over to the car for my approval! They bought a few, and we went on to the next center. The flowers there were so beautiful, I just had to get out and look at them myself! I was happy and enjoying the time with my daughters. We looked around however, maybe 10 minutes or less, when I began to feel sick. I sat down right on the curb and asked Ali to get the car so I could sit back down in the air conditioning. I put a nitroglycerin tablet under my tongue. Ali pulled the car right up to the curb where I was sitting and I got in. I was a little apprehensive, but not overly worried at that point. My daughters continued to choose the plants I asked for and went into the store to purchase them. They had just gone in the store when I realized I was getting sicker. I popped nitroglycerin # 2 under my tongue. The girls came back, and as they were loading the car, I regretfully told them I was feeling pretty bad, just strange, faint a little, and had angina. They quickly loaded the car and asked me what to do. I was suddenly so out of it I realized I couldn't even give myself my 3rd nitroglycerin, and had to ask my daughter to get the bottle out of my pocket and put it in my mouth! I began to cry, and so did they. My youngest was rubbing my shoulders from the seat behind me, which did help relax me. I began to hyperventilate and I couldn't get my breath. I couldn't stand the idea of getting sick on Mother's Day, or scaring the girls, so I kept saying "Just wait a minute, I think I'll be fine in a minute," inside I was trying to calm myself. I knew the General Hospital was only three blocks down the street and I was trying to decide whether or not to go there—how stupid of me! But, I just didn't want to be sick. Suddenly, everything went black, and as I felt myself losing it, I said "I think you'd better take me on to the hospital." Ali was driving and flew to the nearby emergency room. We pulled up and I was aware again, but felt unable to get out of the car on my own. Ali ran in, and Annie stayed with me. Ali returned with a wheelchair and a nurse. By then, I was more alert and helped myself out of the car into the wheelchair. Thank heavens, I was conscious and able to give history and medical information, because it dawned on me I had not informed my daughters of my medicines, doctors' names or anything! Of course, I went through the same routine as a couple weeks ago; EKG, oxygen, nitroglycerin drip, everything. It's rather blurry to me now, but I remember my overriding thoughts were how bad I felt about "doing this to my kids on mother's day!" I kept thinking, "God if I die, they'll never have a normal Mother's Day again!" Of course, they called their Dad, running to the hospital in a new car, he was test driving because one of our cars had finally died that week! Never enough stress I guess. They decided to send me by ambulance to the regional hospital since my doctors were there. I remember the ambulance ride, but the rest of the week is blurry now. I think they did more tests, adjusted my medicines and sent me home by the end of the week.

That week we talked to many family and friends. One of our friends worked with a cardiologist at the University Hospital, and she volunteered to talk with him about my case, and before I knew it I had an appointment on June 1, 1999 with a cardiologist at University hospital. I was scheduled to return to the local cardiologist here! I returned to cardiac rehabilitation, but had so much angina that they decided I should not return until I saw the doctor and got permission to continue. I arrived at the doctor's office with apprehension to say the least. I had no idea whether to expect just a brief consultation and appointment to return, or told to continue with the doctor back home, or what. What I got was put in the hospital immediately. I was told that a group of cardiologists would review my catherization from April the next morning and make recommendations for the next step. The next morning before 8 a.m. a group of resident's, interns, doctors, etc, came in to tell me they were going to do another catherization, and then do an intervention if possible. I was awake through the procedure, which I found more interesting than scary, since I had good local sedation, and felt secure at one of the best hospitals in the country. I was amazed at what the doctors described to me, and what I could see on the monitor! Everything was blocked, all my arteries! Top to bottom it seemed and most at ninety five percent or more, and they said there were multiple small vessel blockages. They were able to angioplasty two blockages and install two stents in my left circumflex artery that morning. Afterwards, I had my first MAJOR chest pains! The pain made me lift myself off the bed, level 9 and 10 on a 10-point scale! I was scared and sick! They went back in and did another catherization, to see if the stents had slipped or anything, they were fine. I do not know why, I had so much pain. I spent five shocking days in the hospital, shocking in that I began to understand the seriousness of my illness for the first time. I actually heard the word "transplant" applied to me for the first time. I learned that because my arteries were too small, and the blockages too diffuse (severe, top to bottom), I was not eligible for a bypass. That is how most people regain some circulation in their heart. My husband and I were "counseled" for several hours on different new or experimental possibilities for treatment. After further testing, however, I was disqualified for all but possibly a heart transplant or a new surgery called transmyocardial revascularization (TMR), which I will explain later. I easily chose the TMR, and came home to wait to see if my insurance company would approve it for me. I then wait for a randomized assignment from the national clearing house as to when, I could have it, sometime between immediately and September probably!

How could I ever explain how I felt when I came home? I was sick, scared, amazed, depressed, and afraid I'd have a heart attack and die. I'd been told I was at very high risk for the heart attack that, I still had apparently not ever had to everyone's amazement! I was worried that I'd never go to work again and what would we do financially, would we lose our new house? How would we send our youngest to college? But most of all, I worried about my husband. He'd been so wonderful, so supportive, and being in a new job himself, he had no time off and had to take the time with me off without pay. He was doing all the cooking, cleaning, and laundry that was done in the house. Our youngest daughter was away for the summer, on her special trip to Europe, planned long before I got sick. She then was to go to Governor's School, a special honor for academically gifted students. I was very isolated, unable to get out of the house, after years of working and being an active volunteer in my church and community before moving down to Eastern North Carolina recently. I was very depressed. Max had watched his mother take care of his invalid, wheelchair-bound father who had multiple sclerosis. I couldn't stand the thought that he might end up caring for me the same way! We had both watched his mother suffer in the caretaker roll, and die before his father, who then had lived with us until his death. I wanted Max to leave me, to divorce me, I was distraught and hurt and angry. A part of me wanted just to die, and get it over with. I didn't want my family to watch me get sick and die either, I couldn't stand that thought. I was their caretaker, I couldn't take "letting them down." My closest friend of thirty years, Carol in Hawaii, was a constant support on the phone and even came to see me! She had been my college roommate and had introduced me to my husband. She convinced me that it would be more harmful to leave my family than to die with them, if need be. I thought a lot about transplant; could I stand to live knowing someone else had died so I could live? Dear God, I didn't know. It was a hard, hard time. I was sustained by my family, near and far, my minister, friends and coworkers. I was humbled, moved, and uplifted by people praying for me, many that I didn't even know. Former clients who found out I was sick rushed to give me the support I'd tried to give them in their darkest hours. I felt my faith in God increasing tenfold!

The TMR surgery ended up being scheduled for July 14, 1999. I kept focused on that, hopeful that it would be the answer to give me back my life!

I put myself emotionally on hold, took my 13 medicines a day, and waited. I read ravenously, lots of escapist literature. I couldn't sit up straight for very long, so Max moved the computer over to the end table next to the sofa so I could use it in a half reclining position. I learned to e-mail, and Ali and her boyfriend Greg even taught me how to "chat" in a heart disease treatment and support group online! That became my world, the computer and Web-MD. I made friends all over the country, who also had heart disease, younger and older than me, people who really understood the depression, the fear, and the sickness! It kept me hopeful as well, since we talked about new treatments on the horizon as well. But, there was no one there who knew about TMR, or who had had it, and I was lonely for that.

As June moved into July, I knew I was getting sicker, I was weaker, and had angina more often and for longer periods of time. The rule is when you have angina, you put one nitroglycerin under your tongue, wait 5 minutes, and if its not gone away, take another, wait 5 minutes, if its not gone, take a third one then head to the hospital or call the ambulance. That's apparently the national rule, and it had been drilled into my head. However, I'd have had to go to the hospital, a half an hour away, every other day with that rule! Usually I would take 3, five minutes apart, and the angina would recede only to return in forty five minutes to an hour. I'd take three more. I'd learned that it usually finally went away in 3 or 4 hours altogether. I'd take aspirin, take a warm bath, meditate, listen to music, anything to try to stay calm, relax and make the angina go away. The weekend before my surgery, Annie was coming home for a mid-semester break; Ali and Greg were coming also. I was so excited, yet focused on making it to surgery the next week. I knew I was getting sicker and sicker. Here are some notes, from a journal I was keeping at that time:

Journal

Friday, July 9, 1999

Annie is coming home for a two-day break from Governor's school. I've missed her so much and am so excited that she's coming home today. Max left about 5a.m. to drive almost 4 hours to collect her and a friend. I'm trying hard to stay calm. I want us to have a nice weekend; Ali and Greg are coming tomorrow. We'll celebrate Annie's 17th birthday, and try to just have some quiet family time before my TMR surgery next Wednesday. It's been a rough week, with one to two periods of ischemia and angina every evening. I am amazed by how many people are praying for me. All I want right now is a quiet family weekend, and to make it to surgery next Wednesday. Several people with stronger faith than me have said God has told them this will turn out okay. I'm beginning to believe that again, although I was so discouraged a couple weeks ago with the transplant talk. I have already thanked God for the miracle he'll give me next week, as well as constantly for all my many blessings, especially, Max.

2:45 p.m. Geez, it feels like a little ischemia is starting and I'm a little nauseated. I have a little angina, pain level 1. I'll take one nitro-glycerin; it'll go away. Max and Annie will be home soon—deep breaths; be calm.

2:50 p.m. Pain's up to 2, nitroglycerin #2

3:00 p.m.—Max called, they're about 30 minutes away—Halleluia! The chest pain is gone, I just feel weak. I will just keep lying here on the sofa, and try to nap, they'll be here soon, think calm thoughts.

3:30—They got home; it is great! Annie looks happy and great. I felt too weak to even get off the couch and welcome her, but it didn't keep us from having a good hug.

4:00—Pain's back, level 2, take 1 nitroglycerin (3 total)

4:05—Angina, level 1-2, take 1 nitroglycerin. The rule is 3nitros, 5 minutes apart, if the pain isn't stopped go to the hospital. This is my fourth in 80 minutes, let's wait and see if it stops. I just want to make it to next Wednesday.

5:00 p.m.—Yea, I feel better, like I can get off the couch and walk around, and my chest won't scream if I do! I actually get to eat something like soup. Maybe, no fat, I can have just black bean soup.

It seems like things worked out all right. Right!—Wrong!—By 7:00 p.m.is when I realized, I'd let myself become too sick and too weak. I had to ask Max to call the ambulance to take me to the local hospital. That started a nightmare for the next seven days! I went to my local hospital where upon judging my serious instability and knowing I was scheduled to have the TMR surgery the next week, the doctors decided to send me on to the University Hospital. In fact, they were apparently so worried about me, they decided I should be flown there in a helicopter! When I heard that, I got so scared, I thought I would have a heart attack for sure! I begged to be sent by ground if possible (I've never flown in a helicopter) and they agreed to send me by ambulance. I left my local hospital about 2a.m. and arrived at the hospital about 4:30a.m.. I was rushed into intensive cardiac care and given close attention. The goal was to stop the angina, which had been plaguing me since the afternoon before. Instead of trying to retell all the events, I've decided to include a letter I wrote about the experience to my cardiologist at University Hospital afterwards.

July 20, 1999

Dear Doctor ____

I am writing to express some serious concerns, I have about this last week that I spent at the hospital. My hope is that you will think about these, and discuss them with me at my visit to you July 26. My concerns don't actually apply to you personally, but since you are my doctor and I am concerned about the quality and safety of my medical care last week. I'm not sure whom else, if anyone, I should discuss this with. I am also unsure of the ramifications of my stating my objections very specifically, but if you feel angry or defensive, or if your practice has rules we cannot work around, then I will seek help elsewhere, I am not saying I want to do that.

First, let me be clear that, I am not talking about my nursing or staff care. In fact I found that generally excellent and very caring.

One concern, I have centers around the treatment I received when I first arrived there. It was about 4:30 a.m. Saturday morning July 10, and I had been in pain intermittently since 3 p.m. on Friday. I had been at the emergency room at Regional Hospital from 7:30 p.m. Friday to 2:00 a.m. on Saturday. About 11p.m on. Friday night, they administered morphine (maybe it was earlier), and the doctor and a nurse were standing right next to me. I experienced immediate level 10 pain, like an "explosion" in my chest. The nurse said "Oh, my God, we won't do that to you again." I assume I had a bad reaction to the morphine. About, I'm unsure, 8—10 a.m. Saturday at University, a young intern wanted to give me morphine. I told her what had happened, and that morphine and Ativan apparently hype me up instead of calming me down. She totally dismissed that I could possibly know what I was talking about, and responded that she'd never heard of that kind of reaction to morphine, and that it was their policy to give morphine, and she would if she decided to! Excuse me for trying to prevent trouble and help! I responded "If you give me morphine, you and a nurse stand right beside me and be ready to take care of the results." I'm pretty sure she didn't give me morphine. She was actually very compassionate later, when I began to cry out of sheer exhaustion. She was convinced, I was afraid of my upcoming TMR. If anything, I was afraid I had become too unstable to have it; which came to be the case. I wanted that surgery. The lack of respect and belief bothered me. Not just her, but my apparently admitting fellow was down right rude, but he was brief, and appeared asleep, not that that excuses him.

Another, more serious situation occurred after my second catherization on Wednesday, July 14, I believe I had an allergic reaction, perhaps to the contrast medium that was used during that procedure. It began immediately after the procedure, in the recovery room, while a woman was pressing on the femoral artery where the catheter had been inserted. I began to experience rapid, shallow breathing, which I was not consciously able to slow down (I tried). I informed the woman that I had begun not only to feel nervous, but that it felt like "all my nerves were firing," that I was "coming out of my skin." She simply said "I'll get someone to take you up to your room as soon as possible." I was in pain and feeling agitated, and I began to cry. I did not feel scared, or frightened. The symptoms intensified as I reached my room, and my nurse stood beside me observing. The intern may have observed some of it, I am unsure. I know that another entered my room as the symptoms were subsiding (I believe it had lasted 30 to 40 minutes). I have experienced some restlessness and agitation after every catherization. I expected him to suggest some action to provide relief and comfort. Instead I received what I perceived as an angry, almost threatening, certainly disrespectful lecture on the panic attacks and panic disorder I was experiencing. How he "ought to send me to a psychiatrist!" (With his voice raised) It is interesting that in my profession, we do not consider a psychiatric consultation a threat to be uttered, but a helpful suggestion, if needed. Since, during the catherization, the surgeon had also indicated that, since my angioplasty from Monday was still open, that my angina pain had all been in my head. He said "All your level 10 anxiety." I think he is an excellent surgeon, and gave me a great gift on Monday, opening my LAD. However, I experienced him as defensive when it was decided to examine at my angioplasty last June. This time, I felt that he was blaming me somehow, saying that I had done something wrong, and he was fussing at me. Back in my room, he raised his voice as he said, "Where's the JOY you should be displaying?" This was said at the end of his lecture about my having panic disorder as I was just coming out of whatever happened after the catherization. When I suggested, that I thought I had had some type of allergic reaction, he said "Absolutely not" that it was "panic." I reminded him that as a psychologist, I was very familiar with panic disorder and felt no special fear or anxiety during that episode. He completely dismissed me, and I felt giving me the old "histrionic female" label, that some arrogant male doctors still do unfortunately. He then left the room with a parting shot at my husband. He extended his right arm out completely, right over top of me in bed, pointed at my husband, (who had confronted him in the hall about all the panic and anxiety talk) and said "And YOUR anxiety is ten times worse than hers, turned and stomped out of the room! I was incredulous to receive such treatment! Yes, I had been anxious and worried all week, and with good reason I believe. I was in intermittent pain from 3 p.m. Friday, to noon Saturday, I had become too unstable for TMR, and I had talked seriously with the doctor about the heart transplant. I had had surgery I'd been told was impossible just last month, and knew it statistically wouldn't last long. Do you think the doctor helped us in any way? He doesn't know us from Adam, yet he accused us of all kinds of things, when I was simply a very sick patient and my husband was a very scared man. We are actually well known in our community, professionally and personally, as patient, professional, intelligent, calm people. And yes, I realize I do not need to provide references, but you do not know us personally, and I was led to believe we might need to! Bottom line, I never want that doctor "attend" me again. I hope that does not mean that I have to leave your practice, but I must be able to expect respect and trust, and team-work with my doctors. I got none of that from him. Besides that, I think he misjudged my reaction after the catherization Wednesday, and that I had an allergic reaction. I have pulled up several articles on the Internet, and I have consulted several other medical professionals, who all seem to have seen these reactions. I don't understand why it's not being recognized at the hospital. I also think this doctor owes an apology to my husband and me for his "yelling" at us, but I don't expect to get it. I must have your assurance however, that I will never have to depend on his treatment again in your absence, and that I will be given treatment to prevent or quickly treat any similar reaction to catherization in the future.

One more thing, early Wednesday morning, July 14, I believe, I noticed a burning, stinging sensation on the inside of my left leg beside and above my knee, in a pattern towards the puncture for my catherization. I told the nurse and several other staff that it was really bothering me, could something be done, and I felt ignored. I thought it was topical, some other kind of allergic reaction, but I couldn't imagine what. A visiting friend said he'd experienced the kind of burning on the top of his foot after back surgery. His doctor said it had come from the compression of nerves, or the inflammation of the nerve near the surgical sight. They treated his with some type of steroids. When the technician leaned on my catherization wound after the catherization on Wednesday, the burning increased ten fold. I told her, and she responded she'd never heard of that kind of reaction. "You'll be okay." Basically, dismissing me again, and not believing me, since she had just been hearing the surgeon go on about my "anxiety." I assume, she believed that was what was going on. Since returning home, I've read several articles that clearly describe this phenomenon after catherization! Again, why was I ignored? Surely the staff at the hospital knew about this problem. I came home with this still bothering me, and it was badly stinging and burning. It was very irritating, and it has continued through today, though it has decreased in intensity.

I am really worried about this experience, and I want assurance that I will be believed and trusted by my doctors, your partners and interns, in the future. I am afraid because I am emotional and cry sometimes, that I have been "written off" as an anxious female. I only report what is true for me, and what I observe. I feel I cowered under this time, next time I plan to be a lot more assertive, and if I don't get relief, I'll speak up until I do. Someone else will put judgmental labels on me, I'm sure, but it will be worth it to feel better.

I appreciate your time in reading this epistle, and am hopeful for a respectful and supportive response from you.

Sincerely,

Helen Holshouser

As you can tell, my stay at the University Hospital from July 10th to the 15th had not been fun. On Sunday, July 11th, after consulting with the head of the transplant team during the day, I found it impossible to sleep that night. I had sent Max and Ali home or to our friends' house to sleep, but I stayed awake and by 3 a.m. I was quite distraught and in tears. A kind nurse offered to call the chaplain on call, and called the intern on call as well, since I was experiencing some chest pains. Of course at 3 a.m, in a large teaching hospital interns are on call. Immediately a tall, lanky young man, who looked to be my daughter's age came into my room and introduced himself as the intern in charge at that hour. He ordered a "Stat EKG," then did a very interesting thing. He asked if I was a "praying person," and upon my yes response, he pulled some notes out of his pocket and read me one of his favorite Bible verses for when he was having a hard time. After all the "arrogant" scientist doctors I had encountered up until that point, I was amazed and very comforted! I was embarrassed at my continuing tears, and didn't want to "bother" anyone, but the chaplain came anyway. He was another intern who had just started at Divinity School. He was 23 years old, and of a different race than me. I was regretting not asking my husband to stay with me, and couldn't believe this young man could help my miserable, self-pitying self. I couldn't talk, and I knew all I would do was cry, so I asked him to tell me a little about himself. He began to tell me some problems he'd had as he'd prepared for his exams and graduation from college, just a few weeks earlier. He told me about how he'd felt overwhelmed and distraught, and how he'd called his mother who often prayed for him. She reminded him that his focus was wrong. That he was focusing on his crisis so much, he couldn't see the possibilities, the hope, of the future. I immediately realized that was exactly where I was. I was totally immersed in my fears and uncertainty, and couldn't see the possibilities. I began to refocus, and talked to the young chaplain about my own family and life.

He stayed with me for an hour or more. The two of them helped me more than anyone else, emotionally anyway.

The next morning, Monday, I had another catherization to see what was going on, and since I had given permission the night before to do whatever necessary, the surgeon decided to perform an angioplasty. The one that he had previously said was impossible. He spent three hours opening my left anterior descending (LAD) artery! He explained later that, there was only a forty percent chance of success, so he had been unwilling to do it before. Now, facing transplant, it seemed worth the risk. The surgeon did tell me that he could not promise that the LAD would stay open 24 hours, much less three months, or six months, who knew? But it would help stabilize me, which it did, and allow me to proceed with the TMR if I could stay stable for four to six more weeks. I was thrilled, no heart transplant, but scared. Would I stay stable another month or so, or not? I continued to have pain all week, and as I said in the letter above, they had to perform another catherization that Wednesday, July 14th, to see if the LAD had stayed open, and it was open. That was five catherizations in the last four months, and several angioplasties, and stents, with more to come.

I went home on July 15th, my youngest daughter's 17th birthday, and I was very happy! The TMR surgery was rescheduled for August 25th, and I made it. I had angina even at rest and weakness, but it was controlled with the nitroglycerin patches and oral medicine. Overall, I felt better after the LAD angioplasty than I had in a long time! I didn't go out of the house, except to the doctor, as I hadn't since May, but I was able to get around the house much better and visit with family and friends more comfortably. The computer and my heart friends online became my support group.

As August 25th approached, I tried to stay calm. I had to go to the hospital on August 24th for preoperative planning, and we decided that I would take the hour trip to University Hospital with Ali and a friend in Raleigh on that date. Max would come up after work on the 24th. We couldn't afford the loss of two incomes, and Annie needed to stay in school, which had already started for her. She had been sick and had missed four days of her senior year. With their attendance policy, we thought she should stay home. Once more let me share some journal entries with you.

Tuesday, August 24, 1999, Sandy Irving accompanied me to the hospital. Sandy was such good and supportive company for the long pre-op day. It wasn't hard, a chest x-ray, EKG, meetings with the anesthesiologist, surgeon, the surgical coordinator, and a physician's assistant. Although, I thought, I'd been "counseled" a lot, I learned a few things that day that I hadn't realized before. I realized that they would deflate my left lung, and put me on a respirator, which I was to be prepared to wake up on in intensive care, and they instructed me to try to stay calm, and not panic or fight it. For some reason this scared me the most and I dreaded it. I then had to immediately start an internal dialogue convincing myself that I'd be able to handle it, which included praying for God to help me. I also learned about the drainage tube that would be inserted, and other uncomfortable things. I thought it was to be a 4" incision, below my left breast, between two ribs, however, it was explained that the incision would actually be 8" to 10", underneath, and following the curve of my left breast, between some ribs. Then they would cut the pericardium sac around the heart open, put the heart laser right up to the wall of my heart, and make 10 to 20 or more holes in the wall of my heart. I understood that, I had read enough, and been counseled well. Yes, I knew I could die, or have a heart attack, etc. I knew that I would be in intensive care for 24 to 48 hours and in the hospital five to seven days. The physician's assistant told us it would only be perhaps four days. That I might go home on Saturday. The surgeon said it would be longer. Sandy very kindly called Max several times during the day to update him on what we were learning, and how I was, as we both knew how anxious and upset he'd felt about deciding not to come himself. I had glibly bragged and really thought I could handle this day by myself, and had asked Sandy only to "drop me off at the hospital." By lunchtime, I was exhausted emotionally and phys- ically. I don't know what I would have done without her, because she got my food, and I know I couldn't have managed the cafeteria. I couldn't check into the hotel where we were staying until 3p.m. we were finished by 1:30 p.m., and with pre-op stuff (they'd said plan until 3). We had a leisurely lunch, talked and visited up a storm! At 3 p.m., Sandy drove me across the street door to door service, to the hotel to check-in, and there was a line. It looked like forever to me, because I could never have stood in it, or managed my bags. What had I been thinking? Bless her heart, Sandy stood in line waiting, while I sat off to the side of the crowd. I struck up a conversation with a man sitting at the next table who told me, that low and behold, that he was having the same TMR surgery the next morning. He was to be #1, and had to be there at 6:30 a.m. I would be #2, and didn't have to be there until 10:00 a.m. That was such a leisurely surprise. I'd been told before to prepare, to be here by 5:30 a.m. Actually, the scheduling nurse had said the first one might take longer, and to be prepared to wait until after lunch. My only problem was with fasting after midnight, if my blood sugar fell too low and if the surgery didn't happen until late in the day. He and his wife were in the room right across the hall from my husband and me also. He looked a little older than I Maybe up to 10 years older, and a lot less healthy. I think he said, "he'd had several bypasses." We had a good conversation while waiting, and we agreed to wave at each other in intensive care (hah—naïve was I). However, I never saw him again. The next morning they called us to come in a little early. Apparently, his surgery had been canceled, because of a clotting problem. They hoped to do it later, on another day.

Sandy stayed with me until Max got there about 6:30 p.m. He had left work early finally. This was a relatively new job for him, and he had no leave, and had to take everything off without pay. I had been on leave without pay for four months now, and we didn't know when or if I'd go back to work. Economics is economics, and survival. Sandy had been wonderful to me, although I'd insisted she could go, she sensed my needs and stayed to talk, pray, and read! Sandy went home to her family and I knew her husband would keep Max and Ali occupied during the surgery the next day. They are such special friends, thanks to God for them! Max and I shared a late supper and a close, loving evening. I talked by phone with my daughters, sisters, brothers, and closest friends like Carol in Hawaii. I had a terrific, bolstering written prayer from my friend Joette. I had assurances of prayers from so many, it was incredibly comforting and humbling. Our friend Mary would also join Max and Ali waiting, and we compared last minute notes. I talked with our minister, Pastor Lindblade, and he was waiting for us the next morning. Although I'd begged him not to come so far! He is such a blessing.

Surgery day: Wednesday, August 25, 1999.

I'd talked to Annie by phone last night and this morning, several times. We had decided she should stay home and attend school, as she'd missed 4 days the week before with a virus, and what could she do but wait around? I don't know if that was a good decision or not, and I worried about her being alone and worried. But she wasn't actually alone, lots of friends and neighbors were taking care of her, accompanying her and I knew Max and Ali would keep her well informed during the day. She seemed okay about it, probably better than I was. We had plans, and back up plans, and I knew we could get her there if needed in an emergency! Friend and neighbor, Judy Simmons had offered to bring her, as had others.

Ali arrived at the hotel early on the 25th. I was becoming a nervous wreck, trying to contain it, and wishing I could take a tranquilizer then, instead of waiting for just before surgery! We entered the 3rd floor hospital surgical waiting lobby and found Eric, Mary, then Deane. I hardly had time to say hello and get a hug before they called me back to get prepped. They let Ali stay only a moment, we parted with tears of love and a hug. Max stayed until they made him leave. Then the fun began! I think I was given something to begin calming me down among other things, but my adrenaline was pumping pretty strong. I remember being introduced to lots of nurses, the anesthesiologist resident, and his attending physician, whose name I can't recall right now but which I have. Well, my young resident was very nervous. His hands were shaking. I found myself trying to calm him down. Later, I realized I'd spent the whole time making small talk with them, and soothing and encouraging the young resident who had a terrible time with my thoracic epidural, and with putting two tubes down in my neck to my heart. I'm comforting him, as he is saying, "I can't find the space" and I'm saying, "that hurts", and he's saying "more numbing medicine." Several times he told me, I probably wouldn't remember any of this, but sorry, I do! He couldn't get the neck catheter in, called it a "central" approach and was corrected by his attending supervisor that it was an "anterior" approach. He had to remove the tube at least once from my neck, and stitch up the hole, and try again. I could feel a popping sensation down the side of my neck and into my shoulder. I'm not positive, but I think the attending finally did the neck thing. I heard the resident say something like this, "Why do you always have to observe the hard ones?" I'd even responded how nervous I used to get, when I was a school teacher and my principal would come to observe and formally evaluate me, even though we were close and respected colleagues. Later I thought, "Helen you idiot! You should have been yelling and screaming and insisting the attending take over!" I don't know if I'm a wimp, or nice, but that was my life he was messing with, and he was clearly unprepared. I had gone to a large teaching hospital for just such an opportunity as this brand new surgery that might save me from a heart transplant, and I knew that meant dealing with residents and interns. But the reality of it is a lot scarier, and they're so young, and look like babies. I also knew the residents had just started in July as they do every year, so they were all still pretty inexperienced. I guess this is one good reason not to have been able to have this surgery last month when it was first planned.

Then it happened! I actually had the TMR surgery! Later I wrote this description for my friends online:

DESCRIPTION OF TMR SURGERY

Several of you have expressed an interest in knowing more about the new TMR surgery I had on August 25, 1999. First, I want to thank all of you for your encouragement and support. Feel free to ask questions, although the Lord knows, I'm no expert, just sharing my personal experience. I'd still love to hear from anybody else who's had this, or is considering it. I am 50 years old.

TMR stands for transmyocardial revascularization. It's a fairly new surgical technique for patients like me; that have' blockages too severe and diffuse for bypass or angioplasty. But, it's also for people who've had all the bypasses they can have. There are several qualifying criteria and I'm sure I don't know them all, but you do have to have level 3 or 4 stable angina. Level 4 is angina at rest, but I am unsure about level 3. Yet, you have to be stable enough to control the angina with nitroglycerin or something or they won't operate. They say, that's when they have the most trouble with people having heart attacks following surgery, etc. I was disqualified the first time, I was scheduled back in July because I became so unstable it took three or four days in the hospital to settle me down. Then I had to stay stable for 4 to 6 more weeks. I was glad to make it to surgery this time, as I could feel my angina increasing as the weeks went on, but the angina attacks stayed in control.

For the surgery, they made about an 8" incision under the left breast, then spread my ribs, and deflated my left lung. Of course, this was accompanied, by a respirator, a chest drainage tube, a thoracic epidural, and 2 catheters placed down my neck. The catheters lead to my aorta I believe, to infuse blood quickly if needed it, and one was a swan catheter to monitor for cardiac heart failure signs due to any swelling of the heart that could be caused by the bruising of the laser shots.

The next step was to cut open the sac around my heart. Then they took a heart laser gun, and in my case made 14 holes in the wall of my heart, being careful to avoid the arteries! Thank heavens! They make different numbers of holes for different people, from 10 to 40 I gather, and I didn't really ask why 14? I now know, that I have a lot to ask later! You have to forgive me, I'm only a few days out, and I was a little "out of it" at the time of hospitalization! The laser shot is computer timed with the flow of blood into the heart. They shoot when the heart is full of blood and that stops the laser from going all the way through the heart! The holes they make are like one mm wide I understand. Although this surgery is now FDA approved, and clinical trials are finished, there've been only a thousand or more done in the U.S, and they readily admit they aren't sure exactly how it works, or what the long-term results will be yet. However, it's an alternative before heart transplant for me. My injection fraction is a good, forty nine percent, but all my arteries and many capillaries were blocked, and too much and too small to bypass. When we were first "counseled" in June we were told there was a fifty percent chance it would be helpful. By August 25, it was eighty percent chance that it would help restore my circulation. Scar tissue seals the outside of the holes, but the inside of the "tunnels" stay open, forming channels that are supposed to be like new blood vessels to move blood and oxygen to different parts of the heart.

If I understood correctly, (I wonder what my surgeon would say about this summary, we'll see if I'm brave enough to show it to him!) this could actually replace the need for my arteries-thus revascularizing me. Apparently, this is based on research on alligators and crocks! They apparently don't have arteries on the outside of their hearts, but these tunnels on the inside. We'll see. It is also supposed to stimulate the growth of new blood vessels and capillaries on my heart. I hope so! They warned me that, it is not a "quick fix", in fact, reminded me that my recovery was expected to be very slow, because they actually hurt or "bruised" my heart. Supposedly, it will be three to six months before I can expect results. I'll keep you posted. But, I did talk to another man who'd had the surgery as the 7th person at the hospital. I was 50 some-thing done at this Medical Center. His was over a year ago and he plays golf 4 days a week, at 70 years old and post several bypasses! Did I forget something? Bore you to death? Hope not, hope it's good to hear about new things. By the way, another hospital in my state was doing this as a laser only procedure, and I had the option to try to qualify for that. The FDA has not approved this procedure.It is still in clinical trials, and I heard they'd lost a couple people because the laser, is inserted through the arm or groin and had shot all the way through the heart. They couldn't get in fast enough to fix it! I quickly opted for the open-heart technique! These surgeries and so many other techniques are offering us a lot of, hope. Ask if it is available in your area.

You know, there's also that new angiogenisis or veg-f trials going on. That's where they inject a growth hormone in the heart that stimulates the growth of new blood vessels in the heart to form a natural bypass. Unfortunately, I was disqualified for that procedure because I had some cysts, and they aren't sure yet what else the hormone might make grow. However, the procedure is real exciting and hopeful. Okay, I'll quit; my only solace is that no one had to read this in less they wanted too. Remember, this is my layman's understanding and memory, ask your doctor about it!

That was my "official" account of the surgery, here's a copy of the letter I sent to several close friends about my experience in the hospital after the surgery:

Wednesday, September 1, 1999

Dear Bertha, Good morning!

It's so good to be home! It's hard to believe that one week ago today I was going into open-heart surgery! Ali brought me lots of e-mailed good wishes, and I can't tell you how encouraging they were. It was an experience, personally I hope never to repeat! (New mantra "NO BREAKFAST BISQUIT IS WORTH IT!") I read a couple of Ali's "updating e-mail" including the Wednesday night one saying "Mom's out of surgery, doing well and talking up a storm (surprise, surprise)." Well, guess what, that was a surprise to me! I don't remember Wednesday at all, except the anesthesiology prep for surgery, ouch-a story, for another time", those residents! There should be a law against inexperienced doctors working on such sick people, of course, then, how would we get experienced ones? Dilemmas, dilemmas! Hmmm? I wonder what I talked about so much? Who all was there listening? Just wondering!

They say we're going to get whammed by Hurricane Dennis again today and tomorrow. They're not expecting a lot damage, just possibly high winds and flooding, that could mean power loss, however. I hope not, because I don't want to lose my computer link more than the cool air conditioning! Although, I must admit, the lack of cool air, and I seem to start having labored breathing immediately! Heart conditions are a pain!

I know, I'm whining. Please forgive me. Actually, I'm feeling amazingly, okay for what I went through, it seems! I have a ten inch, not four as previously told, incision that starts on the inside, left center curve of my left breast, and follows the curve of my breast and around towards the back. They say, the dressing there will just dissolve in about two weeks, so I do nothing to it. There is not a lot of pain at the incision, more a dull, deep ache, especially when I breathe deeply, or cough, which we're supposed to do, I gather. Joy! I know, attitude, is everything! Keep those lungs clear! I just want to bitch, bitch, and bitch. I don't know why I'm in such a bad mood. I'm not always. I'm happy to be home, I'm thrilled to have this over with! I'm praying it'll be effective for me, and truly believe it will be in three to six months. I'm not in a lot of pain, just very uncomfortable. I hadn't realized how much I relied on the hospital bed for moving about. Getting in and out of a flat bed isn't easy. Can't roll, can't pull, because it stretches the incision too much. Just lying flat does that, and it's not the most comfortable position, but propping pillows around helps. I feel like a fat turtle stuck on my back! (ooh, that hurts) Sitting is probably the easiest, but only in the right chair. Actually, the right end of the sofa for some reason! But I can't sit up straight or it compresses, or lay completely flat because the incision stretches, ouch! I have no arm muscles for strength. Thank God, I can push up with my thigh muscles, so standing is okay. God forbid if anyone tried to lift me! I'm taking only Advil or Tylenol for pain. They tried a ton of different things, and everything made me throw up! They'd say "Get up and walk around the floor." I'd dutifully go of course, along with my entourage of nurse, or husband, or daughter, and oxygen tank. I was having low oxygen levels, lots of fluid in my body, with labored breathing, IV poles, etc. About half way around the loop, I'd start retching and heaving and shaking, and some nice person would come running with a pan and wheel chair to take me back to bed. About 45 minutes later some resident, intern, nurse, or someone would be in here telling me to get up. I had to move around to get the fluid out and the bowels awake. This explained some of the nausea, they said. I lived on anti-nausea medicine it seemed, which did little good. There is no dignity in a hospital!) More than you wanted to know I'm sure. There's so much I want to tell you, you'll be bored to tears! Lots of stories!

Love you,

Helen

Ahhh, home, and alive, thank you God! I came home to hurricane Dennis, and a few weeks later experienced, hurricane Floyd, the worst in Eastern, North Carolina in 100 years! We survived the storms with only a small amount of damage and power outage. Meanwhile, I moved forward in my recovery, battled an infection in the wound site from my drainage tube, my left lung had fluid and partially collapsed, but everything healed eventually! I stayed in the house except for local doctor visits, becoming depressed and discouraged. But my friends and family picked me up and gave me hope, especially my online buddies Misty and Toni. I was taking fifteen medicines a day, a meal in itself! But I was getting stronger, bit by bit, and having, less angina. On November 11, I returned to my cardiologist and a treadmill stress test went much better than before, and showed 3 walls of my heart moving that had hardly moved before the TMR surgery. I was getting circulation from the tunnels! I was allowed to go home, and restart cardiac rehabilitation, and start going out as I felt possible, and move toward possibly going back to work in January or February! I came home so excited and so full of hope! I started cardiac rehab the next week, and decided I'd better start doing more around the house if I was going to get back to work in a couple months! Perhaps I overdid it, I'm not sure. Did I try to do too much too fast? I felt great, went upstairs in my house for the first time in six months! We were having company for Thanksgiving, and I couldn't stop crying for the sheer joy of being alive! I thought I was getting my life back. Thanksgiving was great. We had elevn people at dinner! I really didn't do all that much, everyone else did, but I was excited, and did much more than I had in a long while. The Sunday morning after Thanksgiving I had my first major "siege" of angina. It is one of those three hours things like I hadn't had since July! It scared me, but I got through it. I went to see my local internist, who takes good care of me, the next week. He did an EKG and blood tests, but said to carry on. I did, but seemed to be sicker and sicker. I had developed Restless Leg Syndrome and it was keeping me up at night more and more. I missed cardiac rehab at least once a week because I felt so bad, with no sleep, angina, and aching legs. Meanwhile, Christmas was coming and I always loved Christmas. I actually went back to church, twice maybe. But as Christmas approached, even the little that I did, ordering from catalogs, not shopping, trying to write Christmas cards, proved almost more than I could do. The week before Christmas I didn't even try to go to Cardiac Rehab, because I felt like I couldn't drive that far. I wasn't able to sleep at all due to the Restless Leg Syndrome. I was beginning to "eat" nitroglycerin again, 12 to 15 a day, as I struggled with 2 and 3 hour bouts of angina. But I just wanted to make it through Christmas I didn't want to go to the hospital, so I didn't call my doctor. And I did enjoy Christmas, it was quiet, but both kids and my husband and Greg were there, I made it through. On Monday the 27th however, I went to see my internist. He was clearly concerned, especially about my early morning bouts of angina, and knew I needed sleep. So he added Klonopin, for the restless legs, and Imdur, slow release nitroglycerin on top of the nitrodur patches, I already wore and the two worked a miracle. I slept, but I didn't return to cardiac rehab because I was too groggy from the medicine. I still felt significantly better. He made an appointment for me with a neurologist whom I saw on January 7, 2000. The neurologist said he thought I also had some peripheral nerve damage due to my diabetes, actually I'd known I had some mild damage from nerve conduction tests several years ago. So he started me on neurontin to help reduce the involuntary leg movements that were driving me crazy!

So, here I am, I went back to Cardiac Rehab yesterday, January 14, but I had to quit halfway through because I had angina. Then I had mild angina off and on all day. By 6 p.m., when I talked to my cardiologist's physician's assistant, I was in tears. It wasn't that the angina was so bad, it was fairly mild, but it kept coming back, and I was just so tired and so discouraged. She said that they had hoped of course that I'd be able to return to work, and that they had tried to encourage me, but that sometimes it just wasn't possible. She expressed my very own thoughts when she said, "Perhaps I was just coming out of denial that this might be my life, up and down, feeling okay, and feeling not okay, not knowing, my health not being very dependable." But I believe, if I just knew (I must have wished for a crystal ball a hundred times!) what was going to happen, even if this is it, if I will never go back to work, I think I'm ready to adjust. I've lived wanting that, hoping for that, now I just want to live, to love my family and friends for as long as I can. So if my activities are limited, that's okay. But there is a scary part to that,— finances. I'm better off than so many, because I'm married to a man who's employed and I have insurance through him. God forbid, if he were to get sick. Without my income, and with my current 17 medicines a day, even with insurance, it's hard. It scares me. I've applied for disability income, but I don't know if I'll be approved for it. And even if I a.m. approved, to be on a fixed income from age 50 on is scary.

I've now been out of work nine months. I would never have believed it. What a journey it has been and continues to be. I have learned a lot about heart disease. Nine months ago I didn't know half of these terms.

Nine months ago I had no idea how quickly and completely a life could change. Nine months ago I didn't know Misty, Toni, Cardiostar, Babs, Spider, Calypso, Pam, Ica, Sparky, Prak, and all the regulars in the heart group online, now they are my friends. That's my life. I know I am better off than so many people are. I'm trying hard to learn to live in the present, I know I'm lucky to be alive, and I'm here to love a lot of people and to receive their love, thank you God.

Helen Youngblood Holshouser

*The following scripture was given to me while in prayer. I had asked my Heavenly Father to give me support and encouragement in my struggle. This is the scripture that was placed on my heart.*

*"Even to your old age and gray hairs I am He, I am He who will sustain you. I have made you and I will carry you; I will sustain you and I will rescue you."*
*Isaiah 46:4*

# Heart Disease, My Companion
## By
## Linda Phillips, R.N.

As the author of this book, I realize how difficult it is to relive the experiences portrayed by the heart patients that contributed to the completion of this project. I am encouraged by the contributions of the people who relay their angel encounters and share the magnificence of God's healing power in our lives.

I'll give a short background of myself, and that will hopefully serve to give the reason to the responses I gave during my long recovery. I will start from beginning. I am a Registered Nurse with 22 years of experience in many areas of nursing. Before my illness, I was actively working full time in nursing as a psychiatric nurse with adolescents. I loved my work and put all my energy into helping these young adults.

I was a widow and a single mom of two wonderful children—or should I say—young adults. My son was working and living on his own. My daughter was in college and living at home with me. She was my best friend, and I hers. Since the death of my spouse in 1989, and we had together carried on our lives with hard work and devotion to our goals. I had also lost my beloved mother one-month after the death of my spouse. Needless to say, this was a traumatic period of my life. This was two, almost three years prior to my heart disease and I thought, resolved to the best of my ability. I was focused on making a living and keeping my daughter in school.

Looking back on the events leading up to that Thursday morning, I realize that my medical care lacked professional competency, as well as compassion and concern from my internist for my well being.

I had visited his office many, many times in the months prior to my ultimate event. On each visit, my blood pressure was spiking with extreme highs and on no visit was it considered normal. I was complaining of extreme tiredness, lack of energy and vague pains in my shoulders and arms. My heart rate was always fast usually measuring 110-120 beats per minute. I was experiencing palpitations that were of a great concern to me. Strange, and atypical? YES, needed intervention? YES. Got investigation? NO. I questioned my care, and I was told that I was just under stress since I was a single mom and I had lost my spouse. At one point, I was placed on a beta blocker for palpitations, without even a resting EKG being done. No cardiac or any other medical work-up was done on me during the 6-8 month period that I went on a regular basis to my internist at a prominent hospital. Since I am a nurse, I recall looking at my physician and stating, "Could I have coronary occlusive disease?" Answer, "No, you're too young".

If I had only pushed my own care and followed with my own instincts of a possible diagnosis, my life would be totally different today. If I had been a man, things would have been different. Now, I am called a difficult patient because I am involved with my medical care. Who cares? At least I am giving myself a fighting chance.

I was working on the unit with another RN who happened to be a friend this February evening in 1993. I was feeling rather low in energy and experiencing left shoulder pain periodically. The pain was intense at times, but as usual I had a job to do. She asked me, "Are you okay?" I knew I was not my best, but I had not been for several months. When the shift was over, I drove home about 1:00 a.m. in the morning. This was my usual time and my shoulder area ached so badly, that all I wanted to do was take some Tylenol and go to bed.

All night I tossed and failed to rest. Around 7 a.m., I heard the door shut downstairs and knew my daughter had left for school.

I continued to lie in my bed, dreading to face another day. I had decided I would call in to work. Upon rising, I sat on the bedside and it hit me with a vengeance. Severe pain across my shoulders that went down both arms and my arms went numb. I began to sweat profusely. An inexpressible feeling of being very ill came over me. I knew in my spirit that I was having a heart attack of gigantic proportion.

Profusely sweating, I called my daughter's voice pager and without even thinking said, "I am having a heart attack, come home." What a terrible thing to hear on your voice pager from your mother. That is how ill I was, and so fast. I then called my son across town and he said, "Mother call 911, and I will meet you at the hospital." Calling 911 had not even occurred to me. I am a nurse, yet it did not even come to mind. I did as he said, I called 911 and told them, "I am a registered nurse and I am having a heart attack." They were wonderful to me. They never questioned my statement, they simply told me what to do and that help was on the way. The person on the phone told me to go downstairs and unlock the door, get the phone, and sit down on the floor and talk to her. She told me when the fire department was there. I was sitting on the floor and never looked up as the emergency people came into the house. When the man came in I said, "You better carry where you are going to carry me, or I am not going to make it there." His reply was, "We are the fire department, the ambulance is driving up now." Oh my God, help me! I knew I was gravely ill.

When the other people came in, I heard someone say, "Do you want to get a strip?" He was speaking of taking an EKG strip right then. Another voice said, "No we don't have time, we gotta go."

I fell in and out of consciousness during the ambulance ride. I recall a Nitro being placed under my tongue, but to no avail. Also the EMT was attempting to start an IV, but to no avail. I do remember clearly arriving at the hospital and the stretcher being removed from the ambulance. I saw several nurses running toward me. The next thing I recall, I was lifted onto the emergency room table. This is when another life event took place. It was one that has made a profound impact on my life and my relationship with my God.

As I lay there looking up at to at least 6 strange faces, none of them I knew, I felt alone. The brightest white light imaginable filled the room. The pain was gone and a feeling of peace filled my soul. No fear, only a profound sense that my spirit knew or understood what was happening to me. I looked into the face of the strangers and calmly stated, "Well, I am leaving you now." That is just what I did. They call it full code blue on television. God is real, God does send his angels, and I knew it at this moment without a doubt that I was dying. I had a peace about me that passes all understanding even though I was alone in that room with strangers.

First, my peripheral vision began to close like the aperture on a camera closes. Then my vision slowly came together with the bright light in the middle. When it reached the center of my vision, it then came in toward my face and blackness engulfed me. I can say that I did see a tunnel effect, but I did not travel in a tunnel or anywhere out of my body. I was later told that it was probably because I was resuscitated so fast. The next thing, I remember was that I woke up in the hall on a stretcher with a ventilator, and with tubes every where. My son and daughter were standing by the stretcher crying telling me they loved me.

I was told that an emergency angioplasty was done on me and that I was too ill to survive bypass surgery at that time. I spent many weeks in CCU and the hospital. My kidneys developed a severe infection that caused a high fever and compromised my recovery. For days the doctors suspected and told my children I would not survive this heart attack. It was not expected for days that I would survive this heart attack. I knew in my spirit that I was gravely ill. This is one time in my life when I wished that, I wasn't a nurse.

I kept asking why my fever was so high? I was told that it was because I had a heart attack. Then on the Monday I believe, after the heart attack on Thursday, a wonderful nurse walked in my room. I do not know her name or would not recognize her if I met her but she was wonderful. Her words were, Do I have your permission to call an infectious disease doctor in on your case?" My reply was, "Whatever you and my doctor think?" To tell you the truth at that time I did not even realize who my doctor was. She said, "I am not asking your doctor, your permission is all I need." I have been a cardiac nurse for a long time, and you don't run a fever like this with a heart attack." I gave her my permission and within the hour she had an infectious disease doctor in my room. I credit her for a lot of my success in recovery. Aggressive treatment of my kidneys started and I began to improve. My temperature kept spiking and I kept requesting a bath. That was just a hygiene thing on my part, since I was sweating so much.

All this time my nurse friends were with my children in the CCU waiting room sleeping on the floor, in chairs, wherever. I will always be grateful for my friends, because my children and I had no other family in our city.

I began to improve very slowly, but I was still experiencing sweating at times. One particular night, God intervened. I remember someone bathing my legs. I did not see her face, but heard her voice clearly and plainly. As I was thanking her for bathing me she said to me, "I don't work here, but I told the nurses that if you needed anything I wanted to attend you. The Lord sent me here to tell you that you are going to be all right, but it will take a long time." That was the first time she visited me. She returned two other times and then I did not hear her voice again. Looking back on it all, I believe that I was sent an angelic messenger from God to comfort me in my hour of need. He had already shown Himself to me in the emergency room and now in CCU. I have for the past seven years recalled her voice and felt so comforted that God truly did hear the many prayers of my loved ones and respond to my needs.

The rest of my hospital stay, which lasted almost a month, went as you might expect. Slow, but continued progress with the kidney and heart problem came under excellent care. I was told that, that I would probably need bypass surgery, but that I needed to get stronger first.

After leaving the hospital, I went to cardiac rehab for a monitored exercise program. I had at this time lost over 60 lbs. and was delighted at that; however, that kind of sick weight loss is rarely permanent. I needed to lose weight, but not this way.

On my first day of rehab, I was so weak, that the nurse put me on the treadmill at only one-mile per hour for 3 minutes. Now that is slow! I truly gave it my best shot. I became so depressed with my situation, not knowing what to do with my life and I questioned how I was going to make it now. The death experience had really made a big impression on my life. I was not at that time in the close personal walk with my heavenly Father as I am now. I did not have that to draw upon to help me.

After about two weeks, I began having a tremendous episode of stomach cramps. I could not imagine why? It was not related to eating, not eating or anything I could ease with over the counter antacids, pepto, etc.

My cardiologist referred me to a gastroenterologist for evaluation. She would not do any invasive procedures on me because of my recent heart attack and illness. However, she did order extensive stool tests to see if she could find out what was wrong. Well, she did. I had C-dif colitis from the massive antibiotic therapy in CCU. That is the way you acquire this type of colitis. She wanted me to be admitted to the hospital, but I was not in agreement. I had just gotten out from a stay of a month. This was in late March. You might know that on Friday of the same week, I began running a fever and was admitted to the hospital. My doctor was off and her partner took care of me. He had never seen me and had no idea of what I needed. For the entire weekend, I had stomach cramps and diarrhea. The pain wrenched my gut. The pain medication they gave me was like candy. Finally, after a weekend of severe pain in my rectal area, Monday morning arrive and my regular doctor came to see me. I approached her immediately about my pain. I told her, "You have to do something about this pain, I think I have a hemorrhoid." She examined me and said, "This is not a hemorrhoid, I need to call in a surgeon." What was happening to me now? Had I not been through enough? Within the hour, a lovely older man of compassion entered my room. I was to find out that he was one doctor that did not believe in his patients suffering with pain. He told me that I had a rectal fistula abscess from the colitis and would have to have it drained and repaired by surgery. He also told me that I had no choice because it could get in my blood stream. I could die if he did not take care of it. I would have to spend the night in ICU because of my recent heart attack, but he expected all to go well. I was given a spinal and a drug called Versed. I was told I would not remember anything, and that was the truth.

After the surgery, they gave me enough pain medication to keep me comfortable. I spent a total of 11 days in the hospital with this episode, and the same infectious disease doctor attended me to keep this infection out of my blood stream. This was not a fun time and this type of pain can be very debilitating to say the least.

I went home and continued my cardiac rehab. I continued to have episodes of shoulder pain on exercise. I know the nurses got tired of me asking, "Is there any change in my monitor, my shoulder is hurting." They would cheerfully say, "No." I was scared to death and very depressed. I just could not see my future, only the moment.

It was getting to be May now, and since February I had had an event every month. This was my birthday month, so maybe things would get better. I was still in rehab and doing okay I thought. Not wonderful, but considering what all I had been through, okay. This particular day, we had the cardiologist that was the head of the rehabilitation department and held an open forum for the patients. We were allowed to ask him any questions we wanted to. Since I was a nurse, I bombarded him. He graciously answered my questions. He was unaware that he revealed to me in my heart that my current care could be improved upon. This cardiologist has now been my doctor for the past six years and I would not trade him for the world.

It was late May when I walked into rehab. The watchful eye of one of the nurses asked, "Linda are you feeling Okay?" I said I thought so, "Why do you ask?" She informed me that my face was "puffy." She checked my blood pressure and informed me that we needed to go over to the emergency room and get a check-up. She frightened me and she knew it. She assured me she would stay with me until the doctor came to see me. So off to the emergency room we went. They immediately went into what I call the cardiac mode. All the necessary equipment put into place. The usual monitor pads were placed on my chest, an IV inserted, oxygen by nasal cannula, blood drawn for enzymes, everything in a matter of minutes. Now I was scared, "Call my daughter" were my next words to the nurse. It took several hours as usual for the doctor to tell me what was going on with me. After all, I was not in pain or anything. When he came in, he calmly told me that he needed to do a cardiac catherization the next day. My heart was under an unacceptable load and he needed to know why. Of course, my nerves went to pieces. I had endured such a long road and I was so tired. I had no choice but to agree. The catherization the next day was no picnic but it was uneventful. He told me he had sent my films to a surgeon for evaluation. I knew then that there was no turning back.

The surgeon came to my room the next morning and told me what I needed. He needed to do a triple bypass immediately. My angioplasty in February was now ninety percent blocked. I had had my heart attack in the LAD and it was restenosing. This was a no win situation for me. Surgery was my only option. Depression has set in big time now. Now I had to face the possibility of leaving my children without a mother. There were no relatives my children felt particularly close to who could support them emotionally. My daughter and I switched roles. She became the mother and I became the child. How she kept her grades up, I do not know. We really had a guardian angel, and I just did not realize how active this angel was working on our behalf. The horror of leaving my children and taking that stretcher ride to surgery was more than I could stand. The thought that I may never see them again filled me with fear. Let me explain. I had no other family with me or for the emotional support of my children. For all practical purposes, we were facing this alone in the physical sense. Yet, God had his hand right on top of this situation and I didn't know it. I explained to the doctor who was to put me to sleep that I did not want to leave my room awake. That was an important request and meant the world to me. He kept his word. Three shots at 5:30 a.m., and I was out of it. I had already made my peace and told God it was just He and I and I trusted Him.

I woke up in CCU with the usual ventilator, and all the other tubes necessary for my care. I had come through the surgery and was hopefully on my way to recovery. Instead of a triple bypass, I was the owner of a quintuple bypass. The surgery was not as bad as I had feared. I had a lot of pain, but was relieved by medication. Breathing exercises and coughing were the worst. I cannot say that it was uneventful, because it was not. I still had a long way to go and I knew it. My depression was worse than ever at this point. My doctor tried to get me to take an anti-depressant, but I refused. Don't ask me why, because I don't know. His words were "Linda you can feel the gloom when you walk in the room." That should have made an impression but it didn't.

I was discharged four days later to go home. I had enough built up leave time at work that I was still getting my salary. If it wasn't for that income, I don't know what would have happened to us. After being at home for about a week, I was still having pain in my incision site. The normal course of any surgery is that you slowly begin to improve progressively on a daily basis. This was not the case for me. I was continuing to get more and more pain in this area. I went back to the surgeon for my two-week post-op checkup. I told him of the pain that I experienced and he did not seem concerned. He gave me a prescription for Tylox, a strong pain medication and sent me home. The next four days were horrible, because I could not sleep due to the pain, and nothing I did help me. I would pile pillows up so I could doze sitting up at night.

I called and made an appointment to see the surgeon again. When I went, he looked at the area and told me, "You just have a low pain threshold." I quickly informed him that he had no idea about my pain threshold and that I needed help. He had his nurse make an appointment with the pain clinic located in the hospital. What did they do? They injected my incision site with cortisone. Yes, that was the beginning of the next nightmare.

The pain did get a little better temporarily. Then, the first thing I noticed was a large "pimple filled with fluid" at the top of my scar. Since I am a nurse I knew what it was. I broke down and begged God to help me. I knew that I was now facing another scary monster in my life. I almost decided to not call the doctor and just let happen what was going to happen. It took me about an hour to call and talk to the nurse. She told me that the doctor would meet me in the emergency room immediately. My daughter took me to the emergency room. By this time, you could see the wear on her face. She had been through so much with me. At the emergency room, he lanced the site without any numbing medication at all. The emergency room nurse commented that she did not know how I was standing the pain of the treatment. I do, because I fixed my eyes directly on the surgeon's eyes and never let his gaze go. They did a swab culture and it was Staph. Staph can be a potentially deadly problem unless it is treated aggressively. He put a band-aid on it, and gave me an antibiotic medication. He told me to see him in week.

This was in June. It was another, month, another event. As we left the emergency room, the infectious disease doctor that had treated me on two other occasions was entering the hospital. He looked at me in surprise and asked me "What was I doing there?" as he noticed the band aide on my chest. I told him and he looked me in the eyes and told me to call him if I needed him.

The next week, I took the medication but was not improving. I felt feverish and lethargic and knew that I was not getting better. I looked into the beautiful eyes of my loving daughter and told her, "Your mother is going to die if she doesn't get someone to help her." She reminded me what the infectious doctor had said. I called him and he saw me that very afternoon. I did not realize just how ill I was at the time. In his office, I had a fever of 102 degrees and he took his two gloved fingers and expressed large amounts of pus from my chest.

He called my surgeon and put me on the surgical schedule for the following day. I began to cry. My only thought was NO MORE. This doctor knew me very well, and how I was justified in my feelings? He would not let me go home because he knew I probably would not come back.

The admission was so very difficult. His nurse personally escorted me to the hospital. The next day I had surgery, to clean out the infection in my chest. They left the incision open, and there I lay with this large hole in my chest. It was packed with dressing that had to be changed every morning and night. Of course, I was given with a shot of morphine early in the morning to prepare me to change my dressing. I had such bad veins by now, the IV team told me they would dread a call from my room to start or change my IV. This went on for eleven days. My infectious disease doctor had left on vacation three days after my admission, so my surgeon was in charge. After eleven days of this, I was then sent home, to be attended by home health nurses to change my dressings. I was placed on massive oral antibiotics for several weeks.

All the details of this may seem mundane for this story, but this was a really trying time for me. I cried a lot. The depression was unbelievable! Somehow, I felt that someone else was living my life—not me. It all seemed like I was watching a play, instead of playing the main character. As August approached, my recovery was slow. According to my doctors, I did not need my antibiotics anymore, but the nurses still had to come for my dressing changes. The healing process was very slow, and it was painful to change the dressings.

My father was very ill in another state and I was told that I needed to try to see him or else I might never see him again. I begged my doctor to let me go to Mississippi to see him. I had the nurses show me how to change my own dressings. My father had been bed ridden for over a year and my doctor did not want me around his care anymore than necessary. I stayed with a friend in an adjacent town. I spent the days with Daddy and the nights with my friend.

This particular Saturday, I was tired and decided not to go to Daddy's house. I had planned to stay in Mississippi for a month or so to give my daughter a break. She really needed it; she was so young to be the mother of a 50-year-old woman.

My friend and her husband had an argument that day and it was very stressful at the house. I began to have a very rapid heartbeat which, I attributed to the discord in the house. I went in the bedroom to lie down about 3 p.m. but by 7 p.m., I wasn't improved so I took a Valium hoping that it would slow my heart rate down. At 10 p.m., I went into the kitchen and told my friend I thought I was in trouble and needed to call a doctor. I had remembered a doctor that had treated my dad years before. His partner that was taking his calls talked with me and told me to come to the emergency room. I had not mentioned the infection in my chest because I thought it was my heart causing the problem. When I got to the emergency room, I had a fever of 103 degrees, yet I did not realize I had a temperature. That was why my heart was racing so rapidly. When he walked in he noticed the dressing on my chest and said, "What's this about?" I told him, and he asked if I had a bone scan. I said I had a CT scan when I was hospitalized. He said, "Not good enough." You must realize that this is not a large metropolitan hospital. However, it proved to be a great hospital for my care. He called the people on call to come in at 12:30 a.m. to do a bone scan. I was admitted and placed on painkillers and IV antibiotics. The next morning, he came in and told me my options. I had severe sternal osteomyletitis. The staph infection had moved to the bones in my chest. I had not been cured, just helped by all the other care I was given, and now it had returned. That was the reason for the chest pain, and the fever. I needed aggressive treatment. The immediate danger was that the infection could enter my blood stream and cause my death. They were doing blood cultures every two hours to check for this out.

By this time, I was numb and God had taken over my fear. I faced my depression, and I had a sense of peace for whatever was to happen.

My IV's kept coming out and they decided to put in a groshen catheter in my heart to give me a direct line for antibiotics. I had to go to surgery for this. If not for friends, I don't know what I would have done. I was alone. My children were back in another state. My daughter was in finals, so I did not even tell her.

The day they took me to surgery, I was totally alone in my plight. God was my companion. By now, this has become humorous. When the young man with that dreaded stretcher came to get me, I sat up on the stretcher and did not lie down. I had him stop by the nurse's desk. I sat on the stretcher in that lovely hospital gown with my back shining for all to see. I handed my expensive jewelry to the nurses and told them if I died, to "tag my toe" and give my jewelry to my children.

In the surgery holding area, I told the doctor that if he had any Versed in that room I wanted it. That is a drug that puts you in la-la land. He quickly obliged me in my request. I stayed in that hospital for thirteen days, with morning and evening antibiotic infusions, and I slowly improved. I was sent or to my friend's house, only to be visited by home health nurses twice a day. This went on for about two months. I would get up, take my drip bag out of the refrigerator, let it stand to room temperature, and wait on the nurse. Then I would spend the next three hours taking an antibiotic drip. This was repeated at night around 7 p.m. The situation at my friend's house changed, and I went to stay the remainder of my treatment time in the home of my brother. He lived in an another city and all my treatment protocol had to be changed with the nurses. I felt very alone, and my depression is now almost unbearable. I kept this all to myself as best I could, considering the circumstances. One of the home health nurses, Nell, became a life long friend. Her care and involvement in my life was surely sent to me by God.

I have to give credit to this young cardiologist in a small town in Mississippi for saving my life. He diagnosed my problem, and aggressively went to work to get me well. God was gracious in taking my burdens from my shoulders and bearing my yoke for me. He is the most important aspect of my life. I seek him first in all that I do and he directs my path. I have been doing well for the past seven years. Although, He has told me that He would never forsake me, it was put to the test three weeks ago. I was admitted to the hospital with a severe burning in my chest. The old fear returned, and I told Him I could not go through anymore. Well, God is awesome. I had a catherization and all my grafts are open and operating perfectly. My mammy artery graft had closed, because my cardiologist said the surgeon had attached it to the dead area of my heart that was damaged, when I had the massive heart attack. He said that I had lost the graft probably right after my bypass surgery. God has taken care of me and will continue to care for me on my daily walk with Him. All I have to do is to do my best to care for myself. Trust in Him to do what he said He would do and never doubt Him. My physical limitations are due to the damage that I incurred with my heart attack. My quality of life is far from normal, and I miss all the things I used to be able to do. Just to be able to play tennis again or to enjoy a good hike in the woods would seem like Christmas to me. I have adjusted and will continue to tell people that there is life after a heart attack.

I must say to other heart patients that the depression is very real. I was not told what to expect, and I certainly did not know how to cope with it on my own. I go to counseling today for treatment of depression, and it is a daily struggle to accept the changes in my life. I can tell you that without God, the author and finisher of my life and faith I would not be able to make it…at all.

This story is unusual, and certainly not the normal. Use it as I intended when I sat down and relived all of this. That is, to encourage you to take an interest in your own care and to be informed. Listen to your body, because it will tell you when something is wrong. Listen to what your doctors say, and seek second opinions when needed. Medical science is great, but like anything else, not exact.

Linda Phillips, R.N.

*"Who makes his angels winds, and his servants flames of fire.
Are they not all, ministering spirits sent forth to serve, for the sake
of those who are to obtain salvation?"*
*Hebrews: 1:7, 14*

# Introduction:
# God's Celestial Beings Angels

In the process of following God's divine lead in authoring this book, the inspiration to share angel encounters became very strong. During my hospitalization, I experienced the visitation of one of God's angelic messengers. This experience served to encourage me, and reassure me of God's presence in my long fight for recovery. I had always accepted the belief that angels exist and affect all our lives, but had never personally experienced a visitation, or an encounter with one of God's celestial beings. This angel, without a doubt, influenced me then and will always be a large part of my belief system.

The commercialization of angels in pictures, stationary, and in collectibles has soared in recent years. In this area, we must not lose sight of God's purpose for angels. The collection of angelic merchandise is rewarding to the collector, however, the divine purpose is clearly defined in God's word.

God and his angels serve to support, protect, and inform his children in the heavenly, as well as the worldly realm. Angels worship and glorify God. They are involved in our welfare according to the will of God. "Are not all angels ministering spirits sent to serve those who will inherit salvation?" (Hebrews 1:14).

The move of the Holy Spirit has become evident in astounding proportions with the signs and wonders of this age. "Jesus did many other miraculous signs in the presence of his disciples which are not recorded in this book." "But these are written that you may believe that Jesus is the Christ, the Son of God, and that by believing you may have life in his name." (John 22: 30-31). In no other time has God poured out his spirit in such magnificent evidences as the present day. The advent of evangelistic ministering, the focus on the family, the renewal of the spirit placing God at the center of our lives has grown in astronomical proportion. There are but a few cultures of the world that has not been exposed to the Gospel of Jesus Christ. Cultures that for centuries have worshipped idols, spirits of animals, and now been converted by the Holy Spirit in a vast move of faith and acceptance of Jesus Christ as their Lord and Savior.

Among God's signs and wonders is the presence of angels. People of all cultures, educational backgrounds, and undeniable sources of credibility have reported angel encounters. Researchers collect accounts for investigations and are yet to prove that angels do not appear to God's children.

Angels in Biblical scripture are unquestionable. God uses angels through out the Old Testament and the New Testament as messengers, guardians, and protectors. Psalms 34:7 tells us, " The angel of the Lord encamps around those who fear him, and he delivers them." Knowing that God's angels surround and protect me provides a loving feeling of God's presence in my life.

In the hierarchy of the angels as revealed to us in scripture, the greatest and highest are known as the "cherubim," described as having four wings, among whom are the "Four Living Creatures."

"Cherubim with whirling, flaming swords guarded the gate of access back into Eden after Adam and Eve were expelled, to keep them from eating of the Tree of Life in their fallen condition. In other words, they could not return to fellowship with God except by the way of the cross. Two figures of cherubim with outstretched arms covered the mercy seat which sat on the top of the Ark of the Covenant in the Tabernacle of Moses and later in the Temple of Solomon." (Lambert Dolphin)

The Hebrew term Seraphim means literally "Burning Ones." They have a humanlike appearance; hands, faces, feet, etc. and six wings. They have a consuming devotion to God and perform a glorified divine type of service. They are found surrounding God's throne and singing his praises unceasingly.

The scripture depicts the Archangel Michael specifically in Jude 9 and in Daniel 10:13. Michael is called "one of the chief princes." He is the defender of Israel, and fights God's enemies. He is the leader of the angels who remained faithful to God. He overcame Lucifer and the bad angels and cast them out of heaven. St. John speaks of the great conflict at the end of time, which reflects also the battle in heaven at the beginning of time. Many times he has aided those who were faithful to God; he will come to the aid of the faithful.

Gabriel, God's messenger moves swiftly to carry out God's commands. Gabriel is recorded as flying swiftly to Daniel's side. (Daniel 9:21) The angel Gabriel, whose name means "Power of God" appeared to the prophet Daniel, and to Zachary to announce the forthcoming birth of John the Baptist (Luke 1:11, 19). Gabriel appeared to the Virgin Mary to announce the birth of Jesus (Luke 1:26). Gabriel is mentioned twice in the New Testament, it is Gabriel that provided strength to Jesus in the garden. In the Christian tradition, Gabriel is the angel of Mercy, while Michael is the angel of judgment.

Gabriel in his own words, " I am Gabriel, who stands before God" (Luke 1:19). This leads us to believe that they are among the highest of God's messengers.

Angels are spirit beings; they do not possess fleshy bodies. At times, they can appear on Earth in human form. "Do not forget to entertain strangers, for by so doing some people have entertained angels without knowing it."(Hebrews 13:2). God has supplied our needs through his Grace and Mercy. In his word, God has told us that his angels are sent to comfort us, support us, and protect us even when we are of angelic presence.

In Hebrews 13: 5 God's word reassures us that he will:

"Never will I leave you;

Never will I forsake you."

"So we say with confidence,

"The Lord is my helper; I will not be afraid, What can man do to me?"

The inclusion of angel experiences in this book is to support and encourage heart patients. God in his wisdom will always be there for us, to support us, to bless us according to his will for our lives.

He reminds us daily of his presence in many ways. We are always entertaining angels yet may be unaware of the angelic presence. We need to strive for the sensitivity to hear God's voice, as God tells us. "Whether you turn to the right or to the left, your ears will hear a voice behind you, saying, "This is the way; walk in it." (Isaiah 30:21) The people that lived these angel encounters submitted their experiences to me. I did not alter them. They are given in the spirit of encouragement and hope for anyone that needs the touch of an angel.

# Angelic Research

By
Emma Heathcote
Department of Theology
University of Birmingham, UK.

The word 'angel' is derived from the Greek, translated from the Hebrew meaning 'messenger'. This literal meaning of the word indicates the angel's primary function within scripture, is that of divine emissary and mouthpiece for God's will. Although all of the angels mentioned in the scriptures are male, depictions of angels within art almost always depict females. This is likely an attempt to convey the beauty inherent in the concept of the angelic being. It is also true that while referred to as a male, the angels are traditionally regarded as asexual and therefore often seen as having an effeminate radiance, setting this divine beauty apart form mortal beauty. There are, in Christian tradition, nine orders within the angelic hierarchy. In order of importance they are Seraphim, Cherubim, Thrones, Dominations, Virtues, Powers, Principalities, Archangels, and Angels.

Seraphim: From the Hebrew meaning 'Burning Ones'. The seraphim are referred to in a vision by the Hebrew prophet Isaiah (Isaiah 6:2-6), these six-winged beings surround the divine throne and praise God, they are the highest of the angelic orders.

Cherubim: In ancient Hebrew, the cherubim are thought to be animal in nature, taking the form of winged beasts. God placed them at the East Side of Eden to prevent humans re-entering the garden (Genesis 3:24). They also function as God's chariot (Psalms 80:1, 18:10). Often depicted as winged infants, the cherubim owe this particular interpretation to Ezekiel 1:4-28, Little is given by way of description for Thrones, Dominations, Virtues, Powers or Principalities. However there are several Archangels who appear throughout scripture and are referred to by name.

They are Michael, Gabriel, Uriel and Raphael.

From the Hebrew meaning 'who is like God?' Michael is traditionally regarded as the leader of the angelic armies. He is mentioned in both New and Old Testaments. According to both the book of Revelation and the apocryphal book of Enoch Michael led the heavenly armies against Satan and his followers, driving them from heaven.

In the East, Michael or Saint Michael is venerated as patron of the sick, in the West however he is held as the patron of soldiers.

From the Hebrew meaning, 'hero of God', Gabriel also appears in both New and Old Testaments. In the book of Luke, he visits Mary, the mother of Jesus, and in the book of Daniel, it is Gabriel who interprets the hero's dreams.

Uriel appears in 1 Enoch as the one who bound Azazel and cast him down.

Raphael is the angelic healer, the bringer of health and happiness.

Angels: God's motorcycle couriers. No request from the Almighty is turned down. Usually they are invisible, and often turn up just when you need one, but you don't usually realize they were there until they aren't. I began the work with an open mind, not sure what to believe. But now, after receiving over 400 letters, all outlining personal angelic experiences, I find myself unable to be so skeptical. Each of the individual accounts are so thought provoking, there are so many similarities holding them all together, and the majority of them seem to have common situational factors. Maybe preventing a fatal accident, giving a message, appearing at nighttime, comforting the lonely and so on.

It would be impossible, I believe, to read all of the letters that I have received and still remain totally closed to the possibility that they could be true. Admittedly, many could have possible alternative explanations. For example, psychological or even medical, however, there are many which seemingly defy all explanation. I particularly like to concentrate on children's experience, and experiences, which simultaneously happen to more than one person at the same time, having more than one witness naturally gives the account more credibility, and makes it easier for skeptics to accept.

I have spoken to many psychologists at length and agree with much that is said in that field with regard to possible explanations/causes of an experience. However, some stories told by multiple witnesses are often difficult to so easily dismiss. An example:

A gentleman was in hospital accompanied by his two young sons. They all sat around his seriously ill wife's bed. She was on a ventilator and it was uncertain whether she would actually pull through. Behind the iron bars at the head of her bed, the gentleman saw what he thought to be an angel, standing behind the bed. One of his sons turned to him and said, "Dad, can you see that figure behind the bed," and before he could reply his younger son said, "it's an angel!" At this point the, Ward Sister walked over, they turned to her and asked, "apart from us, can you see anyone else around the bed." "Oh my goodness!" she exclaimed, "there is an angel."

This is far more difficult to write off as mass hysteria, grief, stress, hallucination, etc. Each of the people independently saw what they believed to be an angel? The idea was in no way pressed upon them, nor were they a particularly religious family. From that moment on, the woman began to make a recovery.

Another experience I would like to leave you with is this…an account from Lloyd Glen, which occurred in the summer of 1994. The account's is quite long, but please try not to let that put you off.

On July 22nd, I was enroute to Washington, D.C. for a business trip. It was all so very ordinary, until we landed in Denver for a plane change. As I collected my belongings from the overhead bin, an announcement was made for Mr. Lloyd Glenn to see the United Customer Service Representative immediately. I thought nothing of it until I reached the door to leave the plane, and I heard a gentleman asking every male are you Mr. Glenn. At this point, I knew something was wrong and my heart sunk. When I got off the plane, a solemn-faced young man came toward me and said, "Mr. Glenn, there is an emergency at your home. I do not know what the emergency is, or who is involved, but I will take you to the phone so you can call the hospital." My heart was now pounding, but the will to be calm took over.

Woodenly, I followed this stranger to the distant telephone where I called the number he gave me for the Mission Hospital. My call was put through to the trauma center where I learned that my three-year old son had been trapped underneath the automatic garage door for several minutes, and that when my wife had found him, he was dead. A neighbor, who is a doctor, had performed CPR, and the paramedics had continued the treatment as Brian was transported to the hospital.

By the time of my call, Brian was revived and they believed he would live, but they did not know how much damage had been done to his brain, nor to his heart. They explained that the door had completely closed on his little sternum, right over his heart. He had been severely crushed. After speaking with the medical staff, my wife sounded worried but not hysterical, and I took comfort in her calmness. The return flight seemed to last forever, but finally I arrived at the hospital, six hours after the garage door had come down. When I walked into the intensive care unit, nothing could have prepared me to see my little son lying so still on a great big bed with tubes and monitors everywhere.

He was on a respirator. I glanced at my wife who stood by his side. It was like a terrible dream. I was filled in with the details and given a guarded prognosis. Brian was going to live, and the preliminary tests indicated that his heart was okay. That was two miracles, in themselves.

Only time would tell if his brain received any damage.

Throughout the seemingly endless hours, my wife was calm. She felt that Brian would eventually be all right. I hung on to her words and faith like a lifeline. All that night and the next day, Brian remained unconscious. It seemed like forever since I had left for my business trip the day before. Finally, at two o'clock that afternoon, our son regained consciousness and sat up uttering the most beautiful words I have ever heard spoken. He said, "Daddy, hold me" and he reached for me with his little arms.

By the next day, he was pronounced as having no neurological or physical deficits and the story of his miraculous survival spread throughout the hospital. You cannot imagine our gratitude and joy.

As we took Brian home, we felt a unique reverence for the life and love of our Heavenly Father that comes to those who brush death so closely. In the days that followed, there was a special spirit about our home. Our two older children were much closer to their little brother.

My wife and I were much closer to each other, and all of us were very close as a whole family. Life took on a less stressful pace. Perspective seemed to be more focused, and balance much easier to gain and maintain. We felt deeply blessed. Our gratitude was truly profound.

Almost a month later, to the day, of the accident, Brian awoke from his afternoon nap and said, "Sit down, Mommy, I have something to tell you." At this time in his life, Brian usually spoke in small phrases; so to say a large sentence surprised my wife. She sat down with him on his bed and he began his sacred and remarkable story.

"Do you remember when I got stuck under the garage door? Well, it was so heavy and it hurt really badly. I called to you, but you couldn't hear me. I started to cry, but then it hurt too badly. And then the 'birdies' came."

"The birdies?" my wife asked, puzzled. "Yes," he replied. "The 'birdies' made a whooshing sound and flew into the garage. They took care of me."

"They did?"

"Yes, he said." "One of the 'birdies' came and got you and she came to tell you I got stuck under the door."

A sweet reverent feeling filled the room. The spirit was so strong and yet lighter than air. My wife realized that a three-year old had no concept of death and spirits, so he was referring to the beings who came to him from beyond as 'birdies' because they were up in the air like birds that fly.

"What did the birdies look like?" she asked.

Brian answered. "They were so beautiful. They were dressed in white—all white. Some of them had green and white. But some of them had on just white."

"Did they say anything?" "Yes" he answered. "They told me the baby would be all right."

"What baby?" And Brian answered, "The baby laying on the garage floor." He went on, "You came out and opened the garage door and ran to the baby. You told the baby to stay and not leave."

My wife nearly collapsed upon hearing this, for she had indeed gone and knelt beside Brian's body and seeing his crushed chest and unrecognizable features, knowing he was already dead, she looked up around her and whispered, "Don't leave us Brian, please stay if you can."

As she listened to Brian telling her the words she had spoken, she realized that the spirit had left his body and was looking down from above. "Then what happened?" she asked.

"We went on a trip, far, far away." He grew agitated trying to say the things he didn't seem to have the words for. My wife tried to calm him and comfort him, and let him know it would be okay. He struggled with wanting to tell something that was obviously very important to him, but finding the words was difficult.

"We flew so fast up in the air. They're so pretty, Mommy." he added, "And there is lots and lots of 'birdies'." My wife was stunned, and into her mind the sweet comforting spirit enveloped her more soundly, but with urgency she had never known before.

Brian went on to tell her that the 'birdies' had told him that he had to come back and tell everyone about the 'birdies'. He said they brought him back to the house, and that a big fire truck and an ambulance were there. A man was bringing the baby out on a white bed and he tried to tell the man the baby would be okay, but the man couldn't hear him. He said, "Birdies told him he had to go with the ambulance, but they would be near him." They were so pretty and peaceful; he didn't want to come back. And then the bright light came. He said the light was so bright and so warm and he loved the bright light so much. Someone was in the bright light and put their arms around him and told him, "I love you but you have to go back. You have to play baseball, and tell everyone about the birdies." Then the person in the bright light kissed him and waved bye-bye. Then whoosh, the big sound came and they went into the clouds.

The story went on for an hour. He told us, "the 'birdies' were always with us, but we don't see them because we look with our eyes and we don't hear them because we listen with our ears. But they are always there, and you can only see them in here (and he put his hand over his heart). They whisper the things to help us do what is right because they love us so much." Brian continued, stating "I have a plan, Mommy. You have a plan. Daddy has a plan. Everyone has a plan. We must all live our plan and keep our promises. The birdies' help us to do that because they love us all so much."

In the weeks that followed, he often came to us and told all, or parts of it, again and again. Always the story remained the same. The details were never changed or out of order. A few times he added further bits of information and clarified the message he had already delivered. It never ceased to amaze us how he could tell such detail and speak beyond his ability when he spoke of his 'birdies'.

Everywhere he went, he told complete strangers about the 'birdies'. No one ever looked at him strangely when he did this. Rather, they always get a profound softened look on their face and smile. Needless to say, we have not been the same ever since that day, and I pray we never will be.

In the last few years increasing numbers of people are claiming to have had angel encounters, leading to what many social observers are terming "Angel Phenomena." According to Time magazine, sixty nine percent of American people believe in angels and a staggering forty six percent feel they have a guardian angel. One might ask why this is, some attribute it to pre-millennium fever, others to the fact that a large percentage of our generation has grown up with no religious faith and that angels are simply the manifestation of people's need for spiritual fulfillment.

However, I believe that angels are not a new phenomenon at all, in fact my research shows that a large percentage of people who are writing to me now had their experiences as long as sixty years ago. Others have written to me recounting stories of their parents or grandparents experiences which have been passed on down to them.

Today it does often seem as though tales of supernatural encounters are ten for a penny, and the internet has thousands of experiences concentrating on angels with thousands of people accessing them each day, through this, accounts are distributed and circulated ad infinitum. In addition to this, television programs are more frequently including angelic encounters as well as paranormal magazines and literature (which have become increasingly popular amongst the teenage population). To some extent, while expressing the heightened interest in angels, this would seem to lessen the impact of such stories by desensitizing people to them. However, I believe that despite the broad media coverage such accounts are no more or less potent than those experienced in previous years.

http://www.cherubim.freeserve.co.uk/index.htm
Emma J. Heathcote
Post Graduate Research
Dept. of Theology
University of Birmingham
Edgbaston, Birmingham B15 2TT.
England, UK.

*A friendly smile and a kind gesture can go a long way in someone's life. Phyllis, is thought to be angel by a stranger because of her compassionate heart.*

# Am I an Angel? No, No

I was catching a later flight to St. Louis, then on to Minnesota. A couple of seats over in front and the aisle over sat a very pretty lady. She smiled back at me; I smiled at her noticing her pretty floral dress. The rest of the flight was uneventful, but as I was getting off the plane I noticed her again standing by the prompters seeing what flight she was to take and what gate. I stood by her looking for my gate, and flight number. I commented to her that I had noticed her on the flight to St. Louis and she had on a pretty dress. She said, "Thank you;" I asked what flight she was taking? She said to "Phoenix." I looked and she had a two-hour layover, I also had a two and a half-hour layover and asked her if she would like to go to the cafeteria for something to eat or drink.

She said, "Sure." We introduced ourselves on the way down the ramp, and she told me that her name was "Phyllis." I laughed and said, "My name is Phyllis also." As we sat in the booth, she began telling me that she had been told she was dying of cancer and had less than six months to live. She was on her way to visit her children and grandchildren before she began taking treatment. She then told me that she had never flown before and she had prayed a specific prayer. She was afraid she would get lost in the airport and not be able to find her way to the gate, and didn't know what she was going to do for the two hours she was there. She prayed that someone would meet her at the gate and stay with her until she left the airport. She then asked me "Are you an Angel

God has sent?" No, I assured her I was no angel, but did God use me to answer her prayer? Yes.

Phyllis Murphy

# Cop an Angel, Came to Visit
## By
## W.B. Kimbrell

About 30 years ago, my cousin, Brenda, who was about three at the time, managed to get into my aunt's kitchen where she began pulling out the cutlery drawers. She would step in one drawer and pull out the next step up in the next drawer and so forth until she managed to reach the top of the cabinets.

On one particular day she had once again managed to reach the kitchen and began doing this, when she slipped and fell slamming her head on the floor. She was in bad shape, her skull was shattered, her brain was bruised and she went into a coma.

When my uncle arrived at the hospital, he checked in at the nurses station, and was told that a friend of his had come to visit and had stayed with Brenda all day and that he should still be in the room. My uncle went to the room and no one was there. He spent the night at the hospital and left for work the next morning.

That evening he came back and the same thing happened. The nurse said, "Oh that friend of yours was here again today." My uncle asked if by chance they had gotten a name from this visitor, they said no, they didn't think about it but he should still be in the room. He ran down to the room once again to find no one there.

This went on for over a month until one-day Brenda's condition worsened. Her brain is swollen and they were going to have to perform surgery. My aunt and uncle, along with their pastor went to the hospital chapel, talked and said a prayer. After the surgery, they returned to her room to sit and wait.

All of a sudden they heard her talking, they all jumped up and ran over to her. She was awake looking right at the door saying, "bye man." Everyone asked her who she was talking to? She described a man, said his name, and described him in detail including the clothes he was wearing! When the description was given to the nurses, they confirmed that this was the man they had seen also!

Brenda survived into adulthood with minor brain damage. But to this day, she tells the story of her angel and no one doubts her!

# Jim's Angelic Research

Angels can be executors of God's judgment as in (Gen. 19:1, 12-13) when two angels assisted God in the destruction of Sodom and Gomorrah. They also act as God's messengers, as in the announcement of the birth of Jesus (Luke 2: 8-15).

The Bible clearly shows that angels guard and protect God's people: "The angel of the Lord encamps around those who fear him and he delivers them." (Ps 3:7).

But what about guardian angels, angels sent by God to protect and guide individual believers, the traditional "angel on my shoulder," does he exist? There are several tantalizing biblical passages that seem to indicate that guardian angels do indeed exist.

In (Hebrews. 1:14) we read: "Are not all angels ministering spirits sent to serve those who will inherit salvation?" In (Hebrews. 13:2) we are told: "Do not forget to entertain strangers, for by so doing some people have entertained angels without knowing it." In (Ps 91:11) we read: "For he will command his angels concerning you to guard you in all your ways."

In addition to the strong biblical evidence, I have thus far presented regarding the existence of guardian angels, there are several other forms of evidence that I think make a strong, though perhaps somewhat circumstantial case for their existence. I will present each in turn.

Firstly, I would like to mention the fact that literally thousands of people, from all walks of life, claim to have had "Angel Experiences" in which they have seen, felt or heard there guardian angels. Just look at the proliferation of books, articles and web sites dedicated to personal angel stories. While it is possible that a few of these people may be suffering from delusions or some other psychiatric problems, the vast majority of them appear to be intelligent, honest, down to earth people, not "Fantasy Prone" individuals.

Secondly, I would like to mention the very real phenomenon of "Synchronicity" that seems to surround those who claim to have had angel experiences. For those unfamiliar with the term, synchronicity, it involves the occurrence of coincidental events, far beyond what would ordinarily occur by chance alone. It seems to be a universal component of the classic "Angel Encounter." I myself have experienced this phenomenon a number of times, and it is truly uncanny.

Perhaps, when all is said and done, it all comes down to faith. The more you are willing to believe in angels, the more God will allow them to grace your life. Why would God lend an angel to a non-believer who spends all his time and energy trying to deny God even exists? If you are inclined to believe in angels, then this article may have helped to affirm your beliefs. If you aren't sure what to believe, ask God to send you a guardian angel to grace your life. Things may never be the same.

Angels in a daily Life

Jim

*The experiences of firefighters and other medical personnel have astounding stories to tell. They are daily working with the sick and injured in life and death situations. No profession is more adept to witness the supernatural occurrences of God's grace.*

# A Firefighter's Angelic Visitation
## By
## Jim

I am a firefighter of 23 years. I worked as a paramedic for 16 years and I have seen some strange spiritual things. Especially people seeing angels coming for them and then "Boom" the people die! We used to laugh it off but as we were around it more and more, when people say they see the angels coming for them, we really believe them now! Strange but true!

I bet if you asked emergency workers, they could tell you tales of people seeing light and angels all the time. I have been working on a full arrest (complete cardiac standstill) and the people around are singing and praying and oddly, someone will touch the patient while this is going on and you will hear in the background "Here they come, can you see the light? The angels are coming!" I never saw anything as I was really busy but the people were certain that the angels took the spirit. Who knows, at least the people were satisfied! Also, sometimes the family will say things like "Daddy said he's been talking to the Angels for weeks now and he said they were coming soon." This is usually right after the patient has died. When people say they are going to die, believe them!

So, the Light of Knowledge continues.

# Archangel Michael
# Intercession of Archangel Michael
# The Healing Heart

15 December 1999

I am a very deeply, committed spiritual person. My personal foundation is not of importance in this story, but my message is. I have for many years received messages from angels, seen angels and experienced intercessions, not only in my life, but in the lives of others for whom I have prayed. I believe prayer is very powerful and I humble myself in God's unending love for all of us. This is a story about my father.

In 1987, at the age of 62, my father had a 5 and 1/2-artery heart bypass surgery. His recovery was remarkable and he left the hospital only five days after the operation. In keeping with a healthy lifestyle and daily exercise routine, it has now been twelve years since this surgery. However, in June of 1995, my father began experiencing an irregular heartbeat and angina attacks.

That is when my fervent prayer intercessions began. I would write daily in my journal of the news from his cardiologists and invoked God with many pleas that my father's heart would remain healthy and strong. His cardiologist placed my father on coumadin hoping to stabilize the heartbeat. After three months of taking this medication, a checkup revealed that the coumadin was not working. The next step was to perform an electric shock treatment on his heart. Pre-admission testing was scheduled and performed. My father also had to have an angiogram.

It revealed there was another blocked artery on the back of his heart. This was what was causing the angina pain and could mean another bypass operation would have to be performed after the shock therapy.

As I heard of the news, my prayers became more intense and truly deeper. I prayed for God to send an intercessor to protect my father and bring him through this. On the evening of June 15, 1995 I was sitting on my side patio in deep contemplation. It was 11:07 p.m., and it was a very quiet, beautiful starlit evening. My prayers were strong and exact because I believe that in prayer you need to be very specific. Suddenly, I felt this strong and encompassing presence. It was what someone could relate to as awe and reverence. I felt this peacefulness beginning to fill my heart, my body, my mind and soul. It was as though a heavy burden was about to be lifted from my shoulders. Then came the voice, "Do not fear. I am Michael the Archangel. I have been sent to you by God to help your father. I will stay with him until his heart problems are resolved. And, do not be surprised when you learn he will not need another bypass operation." That message, so short, yet so comforting placed me in an ever-humbling state of grace. I could see Michael in my mind's eye, and his words were not spoken outloud, but in a telepathic-like state. The voice was so powerful and clear, I felt reassured and thanked God for this wonderful message. I believed in the words that were revealed to me and went directly to my journal to write everything that had just taken place. Several weeks later, the tests were scheduled for the heart shock treatment. Prior to the treatment, an EKG was performed as well as an EKG afterwards to determine if the irregular heartbeat has returned to normal.

Also, another angiogram would have to be performed to verify the results of the procedure and to once again check on the condition of the blocked artery. Prior to the shock the EKG still showed an irregular heartbeat but afterwards, his heartbeat returned to normal. Now this is not the miracle!

The angiogram was then performed and the test results revealed the blocked artery in the back of my father's heart was clear and open!

Archangel Michael was true to his words. Heart shock treatment cannot cure a blocked artery, only angioplasty or bypass heart operation. When I received this wonderful news, as written in my journal, I went down on my knees and thanked God and Michael for this wonderful gift. I attribute this miracle to the grace of God and Archangel Michael whom God chose to send protection and healing. It is now December of 1999. My father recently celebrated his 74th birthday and is doing wonderful. He and my step-mom enjoy the summers in Ohio and the winters in Florida. It has been 12 years since his by-pass operation. Normally, these only last ten years, but through faith and prayer and the intercession of beloved Archangel Michael, my dad is also enjoying his children raising his grandchildren! So, as Michael said to me, "Do not fear," trust in these words. And, always believe in the power of prayer.

The miracles of prayer and with today's medical treatments, they go hand in hand.

Donna

# My Angel Story
By
Keith

I would like to share with you an experience I had when my father died that changed my *Faith* to *Belief*. I hope that this story will provide hope and strength for others.

When discovering he had cancer and going through the treatments of chemotherapy and radiation. My father decided that the cure was worse than the disease. When faced with the prospect of prolonging his pain and suffering with further treatments, he decided to return home and let life run its course.

The pain of the cancer was tremendous, and in his last few days he slipped into a coma. During the second day of his coma, I was sitting at his bedside holding his hand. I felt the only thing I could do at this point was to offer an intercessory prayer and call on the promise that Jesus made:

*"Whenever two or more are gathered in my name, I shall be there also."*

As I was saying my prayer, a tremendous feeling of peace came over me. Suddenly all the feelings of sadness, anxiety, and grief flowed out of me. The most wonderful feeling of peace flooded my body. It was the most remarkable feeling and I could feel it coming from the direction of the foot of the bed, like you feel the radiant heat from a stove. I turned, fully expecting to see someone or something there, but there was nothing I could see, only peace literally flooding me. I studied the end of the room closely for what seemed like a long time, and as I turned back to my father, I was surprised to see his eyes open for the first time in a couple of days. He was just looking at me with a peaceful expression and I remember thinking, "Gee Dad, I never noticed how blue your eyes were." And while I was thinking, "What a dumb thing to be thinking at a time like this," my Dad closed his eyes, slipped back into a coma. The feeling of peace seemed to withdraw toward the corner of the room and my father died early the next morning.

I believe I was allowed to share in something quite miraculous and have felt compelled to share my experience with others. What I have taken from this experience is a belief that Jesus will keep his promises if you ask knowledge that there is another life beyond this one, a renewed Christian faith and belief in the power of prayer.

May the Peace of the Lord be always with you.

Keith Chisholm

# Yes, There Are Angels
By
Linda Tilley

Children are the closest to God. This has been belabored for centuries. As we grow older, we become more skeptical of the things around us and things we see, and things we hear. Think back, before you were so jaded, hurt, confused by life and what has happened to you. This story is a true one. It is one that you will find incredibly hard to believe. I wouldn't believe it except it happened to me.

Time and place:

The location is Kansas City in the 1950's. During the post WWII baby boom, it was fashionable to play bridge. My parents loved playing bridge with their friends. Once a week or every other week they would get together with some friends and play.

Sometimes it was just up the street, other times it was across town. In either case, all of us kids would have sort of a slumber party. This particular night we were just up the street from our house. All the kids had been put to bed. My older brother was sleeping in the room with another kid about his age. I was put to bed in the middle bedroom with our friend Michael, about my age of four or five and the baby was in her own room fast asleep in her crib.

When I was very young one of my favorite things to do was to look at the sky. Partly because my dad was a commercial airline pilot, and partly because it was a good way to dream. Watching the clouds during the day, the stars at night. This night, the sky was cloudless. The stars were very brightly shining. The moon was just a quarter moon so you could still see the stars clearly. I lay on the bed nearest to the windows, dreaming little girl dreams, not wanting to go to sleep. This was a problem mother and dad had always had with me, not wanting to go to sleep. I was looking out at the stars, concentrating on their brilliance. Michael was talking to me but I wasn't really listening. One star had caught my attention. It was more brilliant, bigger and more spectacular that all the others. As I watched this gorgeous star it started changing. It seemed like it was growing. Getting bigger with each passing moment, I couldn't take my eyes off of it. It grew bigger, and bigger and bigger until it burst. My eyes not moving, I held my breath for the incredible beauty I was experiencing, lest it all be just a dream. From inside the star, there came forth a brilliant light. Beautifully shaped like a lady. The light was so bright it was hard to determine what I was seeing. But the memory of what I did see has been imprinted in my mind for over forty years. Blue shining garments like a dress. The lady had golden flowing hair. The spectacle did not frighten me, it drew me to continue watching. Her face was the most beautiful, kind, loving face I have ever seen. Her hands graceful and loving. She was completely encased in light. Light more pure than I can even imagine today.

Sometime during this event, I whispered to Michael to come watch. From across the room, he joked that the 'angel' or 'fairy' was there to make all of his toy animals alive. That was when I looked away from the window and listened to what he was saying. That was when I felt fear. To a four or five year old, fear is very real and immediate. The reaction to that fear was to flee. I ran out into the living room and hid behind the couch. The parents, hearing the bedroom door open, came to find me crouching behind the couch and crying. My mother took me in her arms and I tried to tell her what I had seen. My parents have always been more open to the unexplained than some. So telling them of the spectacle was not traumatic for me. They never questioned the validity of the sight. Michael's parents went into check on him. I have to assume that they found nothing out of place. I never did learn what, if anything he told his parents. The event was over. The beautiful woman was gone. Except locked in my memory forever.

Years later, I was visiting Chicago, where Michael and his family had moved too. There was one moment when Michael allowed himself to be in a room alone with me. (Something I hadn't understood until now) I asked him about that night, when we were children. The look on his face, his quick departure from the room told me what I had long wanted to know. He had seen the angel that night so long ago. I was no longer haunted with the thought that it all must have been my imagination. I was finally at peace and could accept what I had seen.

Several years still later, with that vivid memory in my mind. I realized a power within me that can be used to help the hurting, ease the pain, and comfort people I come in contact with. At first I thought it was just an emotional tie that I had with some people. Now I have come to realize it is much more. My life has been one of many, many wrong choices. Yet, I also know that even though these choices seem wrong, they were made for a reason. We all have many 'lessons' to learn in our quest for perfection. This is the one thing that would truly make us closer to God.

During the divorce from my second husband, who was emotionally, mentally and physically abusive, I thought of that night when I was a child. I again asked to be made aware of why I was allowed to see such a vision. I think back now and realize that it was because I needed to have experienced such an event in order to be able to continue my life as I was supposed too.

Although we often let "me" into the decisions we make if we were to just rely on a higher power, the decisions would not have the consequences they do. That is where I find myself today. And yet, somehow I do emphatically know that I am where I am for a reason. A friend needed me as much as I needed a friend.

Linda Tilley

# Mamie

The women in my family are possessed with the ability to "see" things. Things that will happen, and we have "visitations" from members of our family, especially the female members and this usually happens when something significant is going to happen. For instance, my grand-mother, who is now deceased, visited me by my bedside about a month before Joe had his transplant and told me "Linnie—get ready child, it won't be another month before you will be called." It is strange but true. This happened during the Thanksgiving holidays. Joe had his transplant on December 4.

Anyway back to my true angel story.

Joe had his transplant and went into hyper acute rejection. His body totally and completely rejected the lung. His other lung was already nonfunctional from the disease that he had, which was fatal. The doctors told me if the lung did not begin to work on its own within a week or two, that if they could not find another lung, to transplant, that Joe would die because he would have no respiratory capability.

I remember standing outside of ICU (they would not let me go in to see him), watching him receive a blood transfusion and thinking to myself (praying actually), "Please, God, please, please don't take him yet."

To make a long story short, at the head of his bed all of a sudden, after I had been standing there for what seemed a very long time, I was in a trance like state. That is what happens when we "see" during the daytime or when we are awake. His mother, who is deceased, appeared at the head of his hospital bed. She was wearing gauzy, white flowing robe type apparel. She looked absolutely lovely and serene. Her hair was done all nicely and I seem to remember it looked as if she had stardust in her hair. She took both hands, put one on each side of Joe's face and looked straight at me and said, "Daughter, his time has not come yet. We will take care of him.—Worry not.

He is in our care." She looked at me for some time while she stroked her son's face telling me things about her grandchildren, (whom she has never seen), and how proud she was of our family. Then she began to fade slowly…telling me again…"It is not his time… It is not his time…We will take care of him. He is in our hands."

Strange, but very true. This is my favorite angel story. I believe it is true. I believe that Mamie did come down and show herself to me and say those things to me.

Joe did recover…slowly…but he did recover.

I only saw Mamie one more time, the night before he was dismissed from ICU. She just appeared at the head of Joe's bed again. She was touching Joe lightly on the face, giving me the most beautiful, most serene smile—of such utter peace and beauty, and that is the last I have seen of her.

Yes, angels do exist. I believe they can take many forms. I have thought a lot about this since then, especially whether or not to tell anyone about it? But, what better place to tell of my favorite angel story, since its a true life experience?

Let peace be with you.

Namaste

# Angel Stories
## By
## Michelle

Believing in angels is very "in" these days, but as far as I'm concerned, they've been in my life for as long as I can remember. I've always known my Guardian angel exists because I can feel him. Yes, I said "him." I don't know how I know, but I just know. I've never seen him in my waking state, but in my dreams he's always got a cowboy hat and a "cruddy" old brown leather jacket and blue jeans on. His hair is dark, curly and a little long and he's got clear sky-blue eyes. Sometimes he has wings and sometimes he doesn't, but this persona is probably just what my subconscious thinks he looks like anyway. I wanted to put a picture of a male angel in here, but I couldn't find one! I saw a lot of sites where people are also looking for pictures of male angels, so if you happen to be a talented artist, I know a lot of people who would appreciate one. Anyway, my angel has gotten me out of a few scrapes through my life, and I've written about one of them. There are also friend's, family and visitor's brushes with their own angels.

Michelle Bechard—Toth
Ontario, Canada

This is one of my own experiences:

In grade 6 my best friend was Melissa. We lived a block away from each other so we would walk to and from school together. We had to pass through the high school parking lot to reach the walkway to our streets on the way home. Well, one day in January, there was an awful blizzard while we were going home. We couldn't see our hands in front of our faces because of the snow and the wind was whipping it around in all directions. Mel was right behind me when we entered the parking lot. All of a sudden, I felt a hand grab my jacket and pull me back onto the sidewalk. A snowmobile hit my boot and I was being jerked back and it knocked me over. I was in shock for a second and then looked up at Melissa. I said "Thank you for pulling me out of the way, I didn't even see that snowmobile." and she said "I didn't do it. I thought you saw him and jumped back! You nearly knocked me over!" There was nobody else around and she was right behind me, so the only way I can explain it is that it was my angel. I didn't see or hear the snowmobile, but someone DID pull me. I would have been killed for sure, but just ended up with a twisted ankle.

Michelle Bechard-Toth
Ontario, Canada

# Angel Encounter

By

Lina Sorrentino

My name is Lina Sorrentino. I'm 44 years old, and as I reflect back on my life, I recall an incident in my mind that I will never forget as long as I live, it's about my angel. I call him Francis now, but back then he was just some kid. My family and I were on vacation.

We were on our way back to California, and as usual, we would stop in a motel with a pool. We had to have a pool; all of us girls were young and loved to play in the water. I'm the second oldest of four girls. At the time, I was about eight years old. I was the clown, the crazy and funny one, always making faces in the camera, always jumping up and down. I was always hamming it up being cute or, I was getting into trouble. Well, this one particular evening, my parents finally got us all out of the pool and dressed so we could go out and have dinner some where. I distinctly remember my mother saying to me, "Lina, don't go out near the pool, I don't want you to get your nice clothes all wet!" "Yes mother, I won't." As I was saying this, I started walking out the door and of course, I headed straight for the pool. I walked along the edge looking in at my reflection as I passed by. Once in awhile, I would squat down and strum the water with my hand thinking how cool and inviting the water looked. It was about six in the evening and I was the only one there by the pool. I remember this as if it was yesterday. Anyway, I was sitting like a little duck by the edge, I mean the very edge when my tiny white crises-cross sandals slipped over the ledge and in I fell. Down, down to the bottom of the DEEP END. "Oh my God," I thought to myself! This is it Lina. This is how it will end. I can't swim in the deep end. I started to wave my arms up and down and at the same time watching the bubbles coming from my mouth. I was trying to yell for help anyone, someone, please help me, I'm drowning! Just when I felt I couldn't hang on anymore, there was a big splash in the water. It was next to me. I felt these arms grab me and push me up to the surface with the strength of a rocket blast! I was out of the water, and could breathe. I turned to see who my savior was. It was a boy. He was older than I, about thirteen. He was sort of chubby and slightly dumpy looking, but he had such gentle and caring eyes. We just looked at each other not saying a word with our mouths but, talking and understanding everything through our eyes and minds.

Mentally he asked if I was okay now. "Yes" I replied. Thank you and I ran back to the room crying hysterically. My mom was all upset because she told me not to go near the pool. I was trying to tell her that a young boy had saved my life. "Hurry come and ask him, he will tell you it's true." We ran out the door to find this nice boy, but he was nowhere to be found. We asked around to the other guest and no one had ever heard or seen such a person at that motel. Back when it happened, I just thought, oh well, it was just one of those things.

Today I know it was my guardian angel and his name is Francis.

Lina

# Walk With the Angels
## By
## Toni Sweiker

It was a beautiful spring day in May of 1991. I had been feeling so wonderful because I had received Jesus Christ as my Lord and Savior on April 21st. HE washed away all my sins. The whole world seemed sweeter and lighter now. I had a past that was full of pain and nightmares. But now...life was wonderful! I knew my life was going to get better and more wonderful with every passing day.

I had no idea that this day was one that I would remember for eternity! I had decided that since it was so beautiful outside that I would go for a walk. My two little girls, Christina and Marcia were in school. So, put on a light jacket and headed out the door. I grabbed my little walkman tape player so I could have some up-lifting music to listen to as I walked and enjoyed the beautiful day.

As I walked, I noticed how beautiful all the trees and flowers are now. I am blessed that where I live, the neighborhood has such nice foliage growing all around. I could see the LORD in everything that grew all around me as if, for the first time I was seeing these things! I stopped to examine some of the leaves on a plant and could see a cross or a star in every one of them. This excited me and filled me with such Joy! I continued on my walk and began to feel a peace and joy that was SUPERNATURALLY given from above. It was incredible! I was being enveloped by this wonderful warm sensation. I closed my eyes so I could enjoy it more as I continued to walk. I was not even thinking that I was walking down the street blind in the natural sense. Some places along the walk have no sidewalks, so I was at the edge of the street. I had no concern about it at the time. I continued to bask in this glory I was feeling. It was so peaceful and refreshing as I was walking, I became aware that there was someone suddenly at my side, one to my left and one to my right. Still walking with my eyes closed, I was allowed by the GRACE of GOD to see my visitors. There, walking beside me were two of the most BEAUTIFUL creatures I have ever seen! I would say they were about eight feet tall. The one on my right had dark hair while the one on my left had strawberry blonde hair. Their skin was more beautiful then any woman and the glow that emanated from them told me who they were. Their faces were the most beautiful I have ever seen! Their shoulders were very, very broad.

They had wings that I heard "SWISH" as they came up beside me. Their wings were high above their heads and curved down gracefully to their feet. They smiled a most beautiful and joyful smile as they each nodded at me! I was so elated that I felt, if I smiled any harder my face would crack in half! Talk about being "Full of Joy!" I put out both of my hands in order to hold each of their hands; I wanted all I could get out of this experience! I walked this way, all the way down the street feeling as if I was floating on air…never once opening my eyes to see where I was in the natural. I didn't care! I knew I was in BLESSED HANDS! I would estimate that the entire walk with the Angels of the Lord was about twenty minutes long. Near the end of the walk, I felt impressed to open my eyes for a quick second to see what I could see. What I saw was the top of the trees on my street! Then I quickly squeezed my eyes shut! I could see all that was going on around me. Since I was enjoying myself so, I had not noticed a few things. Later I remembered that as I walked with the Angels, there had come by a couple of cars and I could see them and the expression on the drivers faces as they looked puzzled to see me walking with my hands outstretched and eyes closed! What was I doing, I a.m. sure they thought! But, they could not see the angels beside me. When it was over, I was in front of my house on the sidewalk.

This was so very intense and vivid an experience that I will never, ever forget it! GOD loves us so much that HE blesses us in ways that we could not even imagine until

HIS plans unfold. HE is a great and loving Creator. Believe for GOD'S best because HE wants to give it to you!

Joyfully told by,

Toni Sweikert,

A grateful servant of a LOVING CREATOR, I LOVE YOU LORD!

Thank you.

Toni

# Medical Angels

By

Daniel Bostock

I have two stories to relate:

I work as a nurse on a medical-surgical unit. I had an octogenarian male patient one-day with terrible abdominal pain due to gallstones and was facing gall bladder surgery. This gentleman was as kind and as good as they come, as was his family, a wife and daughter. Despite his discomfort, he was outgoing and a very pleasant person. I also knew he had a failing heart, poor lungs, and kidneys whose function was troublesome. Yet surgery was intended, and I felt he would not make it after surgery.

Two days, later the gentleman was transferred from the ICU and still just as upbeat and kind as ever. I enjoyed having him as a patient again. His wife and daughter pulled me aside later and related to me that after surgery the doctors and nurses were afraid Dad was hallucinating. He kept telling the ICU Staff to be careful and not bump into the two Nuns standing at the foot of his bed. The wife and daughter even told dad there weren't any Nuns there. Dad insisted there were and they were dressed in old-fashioned white habits and everyone kept bumping into them. It then dawned on the wife and daughter that dad was seeing angels, and those angels remained at the foot of Dad's bed the entire time he was in the ICU. My patient was discharged two days later in fine condition!

Not too many weeks later, I had a patient who was suffering terribly with Chronic Obstructive Pulmonary Disease (COPD) and each breath was a labor to him. His doctors were at a loss as to how he acquired the disease and why he kept getting worse! This was a man who never smoked nor had exposure of any kind to cause COPD. He told me that an angel walked into his room and spoke with him, and told him to have the doctor's check his liver! My patient insisted that the doctors do so, there is a enzyme produced by the liver that acts as a surfactant in the lungs, helping to remove the everyday impurities we all get from breathing. My patient was found to lack this enzyme, a very rare condition, and not one a doctor might check for. His treatment began to replace that enzyme, and my patient went home feeling better everyday!

# Crystal
By
Shirley Simonds

*I share this true story with you as a testimony to a living God and His living son, Jesus Christ, the Savior. Read it as such and it becomes a story with a very happy ending.*

You need to hear this story. If you know Jesus, you will be affirmed in the kind of complete compassion He can bestow. If you do not know Him, you may very well find the desire to make His acquaintance!

I was raised knowing He was part of life, just as much as breathing. I knew He was always there, even thought there were many times I ignored His presence in order to do things my own way. I realized later that He carried me through many of those times safely. He kept hoping that somewhere along the way, I would fully affirm Him in the right place in my life. He never gave up that someday I would realize that I should live as a testimony for Him, because this life I had was not mine anyway, but His. I married at age 18. Marriage and having a family seemed to be the only goal for me. I was blessed with four very healthy boys. When the youngest was one year old, the head of our household left us on our own. We five made a life of our own and did very well, too. We had good and bad times, joys and sorrows, all the ingredients that make up living. I always compared myself to Charlie Chan...you no. 1 son, no. 2 son etc. My no.2 son, Michael, was the first to find that special one and to be married. That first year of Michael and Brenda's marriage they made me a grandmother. I wasn't all that thrilled by that. A grandmother! Not me! At least not to the point of getting involved! I had been fortunate to get through motherhood, so I did not plan to start over again.

Michael Brian, a beautiful red headed boy, was born August 15, 1977. I laid down the ground rules right away. I told them they were welcome and expected to visit me at times, but the baby would go home with them when they went. If babysitting was needed, that they could hire one. He would not be taught to call me any of those matronly names such as "Granny." He would learn to call me by my given name.

Shortly after Brian's birth, Michael and I had some very serious differences. You might say I "disowned" him. The hurt made my heart very hard and I decided the rift was not repairable forever. He took his little family and moved to another state. I only heard about them through my oldest son, Doug. Even at that I usually changed the subject when he tried to talk about them.

Two years later they moved back into the area close to us. By that time, I had found Wayne and we had gotten married. I was comfortable with things the way they were. Wayne worried about the problems between Michael and myself and urged me to take steps to mend the situation. I would not even consider it. As far as I was concerned, I did not even have a son named Michael.

During this time of separation, a little sister had joined Brian. Crystal Michelle was born July 23, 1979. Wayne and Doug had seen her and just had to tell me about her. I listened, but I made no plans to meet her or renew my short acquaintance with Brian. I had just begun to open up to him in the first few months of his life and had lost him. I was not about to give that situation a chance to happen again, especially when there was a little girl involved. My mother and I had always been so close; I had longed to repeat that experience with a daughter of my own. That was not to be, but now there was a granddaughter. I convinced myself that I didn't want to know her or love her. It would just be a waste of time. We would come to love each other and then just be torn apart. I was sure I was wise in avoiding this trauma.

It was my oldest son, Doug that was to bring the family together again. His incessant pleading for a family reunion wore me out, so I finally agreed. I had very definite reservations about this mending process. I was not sure it would work, but to satisfy Doug I was willing to try. I had to remind myself how forgiving God is to help open my heart. We set the date for November 11,1979.

All the family gathered at my mother's first so they could accompany Michael in coming to our home. He was probably more apprehensive about this meeting than I was. When they arrived, Brian came running, as most little boys do, noisily into the house. It was hard to realize that my first grandchild was already two years old. Mother came in carrying a beautiful three-month-old Crystal and proceeded to try to give her into my arms. I backed away and asked for her not to rush me, to give me just a little more time. Hindsight is so much better than foresight. I hope I never again forget how precious time is, every moment of it.

The day passed and we saw all anger put aside, a family reunited, old loves renewed and new loves started. Crystal found a spot in my life and in my heart. Brian took to me as though he had known me all along. I became "Mema!" I even liked it a little bit.

So we went about the business of life. There were problems at times, of course, for no life is without them. We were at least able to resolve them as they came and still be a family that found lots of love and good times in each other. The next two years seemed to fly by. We let our love for grandchildren grow as it should and also the pleasure we got from them grew also. Now, we were expecting a little brother or sister to join Brian and Crystal.

We always celebrated the baby's birthdays with one party since they were only about two weeks apart. We had a small party as usual on August 1. Crystal had been through a bad time with strep throat shortly before her birthday. She was very happy and energetic as she participated in the party. She was usually a relatively quiet child. We always said that was because Brian never gave her a chance to get a word in. So, in the few days following the party she slipped into listlessness without any of us even catching it.

One Sunday, later in August, Michael brought his entire little family to our home to have dinner and to spend the day. Brenda called my attention to some bruises on little Crystal's legs. They weren't near as puzzling, however, as the ones on her eyelids.

We eliminated the possibilities of falls or scuffles with Brian. It then came to focus in Brenda's mind that Crystal had lost her interest in play and that she sat around and fell asleep quite often. She had just blamed it on tiredness left over by the strep throat. As we put the pieces together, we knew we were facing some other problem. We had no ideas what, but we knew a doctor's visit was necessary to find out.

That next morning, the biggest lightning bolt of our lives hit with full force. Michael called me from the doctor's office. He was crying uncontrollably. I could barely understand as he said, "Mother, Crystal has Leukemia. She is going to die!"

That moment was so fleeting, yet it seemed to last forever. I tried to help Michael get control of his self.

I spoke to him in a very loud and strong tone of voice. "Michael, did the doctor say explicitly She is going to die."

"No mother, but she is so very ill. They are sending us directly to the hospital with her to be seen by a specialist in leukemia in children."

I had to try to give him courage. "Michael, wait before you assume the worst. Just be careful going to the hospital and I will meet you all there."

I will never know how I got to the hospital safely. The only answer I can come up with is the good Lord. It must have been He that got me there to hold close that baby I never wanted to know or love; to share with her parents in this devastating event. We would have to pool our strengths to get through this.

Her condition had worsened incredibly in that short time since they left our house just the day before. When I entered the room and saw her. It took my breath away. Surely this was not our little Crystal our little "peanut" as Wayne had nicknamed her.

Even though she was by nature a quiet child, she was very perceptive for her age. The doctor impressed on us the importance of a normal and happy attitude. She must not draw on our feelings of devastation and fear. Any crying would have to be done out of the room away from her. She had enough to contend with and adjust to as it was. Being in a huge strange place, with so many strangers around her and all of them poking or feeling of her or sticking needles in her. Our only reason for being there, as far as the doctor was concerned, was to ease her fear and support each other.

Naturally, she cried a lot at all they did to her. They blasted her blood with massive doses of very strong medicines as they started the chemotherapy that we hoped would kill this horrible disease that had stricken our lovely golden haired girl.

Sometimes she was just too tired or too weak to cry or to care what they did to her. She tolerated it all so exceptionally well that we began to feel that we were the weak ones.

There were so many needles. Needles to inject chemotherapy drugs, needles for blood tests, for intravenous feeding, for spinal taps, for bone marrow. They became the most hated part of it all.

In three weeks remission was achieved and the doctor let Crystal's mother and father take her home.

Michael and Brenda had be having some serious troubles with their marriage. Now the emotional devastation brought on by Crystal's very serious illness only fueled the fire. Each one of them turned into themselves instead of to each other or to God. They decided to separate.

About the first of October, Crystal had to return to the hospital for more specialized treatments. While she was there, Brenda stayed with her constantly as she had during the first stay. Although Crystal loved and needed all of us, she and Mommy had a special bond between them. She had more need for Mommy than anyone else. During this stay, Brenda had to leave her for a day and pay a visit to the maternity ward. It was time for the new baby. I had contemplated this business of another baby coming, trying to second-guess God's plan, I guess. Before Crystal became ill, I had predicted a boy. After she took sick, I prayed it would be a boy. I felt that if it were a girl, it would be an "early replacement" for Crystal. I could not shake the feeling that it would be a sign that we would not be able to keep her. I still believe this perception was a " slight insight from God," one of many that we would experience.

Amanda Lynn arrived on October 5, 1981. She was a beautiful and healthy baby girl. Since she was a very healthy baby, the doctor released her for the hospital the day after her birth. She went home to Brenda's mother. Crystal needed her Mommy so much more that a little Amanda.

When time came again for the release from the hospital, all the little family reunited. My hopes were high for a permanent reconciliation. But that was not to be. If Michael and Brenda could have only had the presence of mind to turn to God or to seek professional counseling, but that is one of life's big "ifs." There seemed to be no way to help or counsel either of them, nothing was acceptable. Stress, raw nerves, inability to cope, depression, guilt complexes; all of that together just blew everything apart. They separated that time and it was permanent. Their only confidence was in their own ability to "get their heads straight." Both were emotionally, physically and financially wiped out. They felt the pressing need of time alone, away from everyone, even the children.

This is when God took a "giant step" into my life and showed their "never going to be a babysitting grandmother" who is supreme in such decisions! I do say that lovingly. He always knows what He is doing and Why?

Wayne and I decided we should take the children to live with us for the time being. I did not know how we were going to make it, I just knew we had to try. I felt 'hard-pressed' to do this business without realizing till later that it was an assignment from God. It came at a time when Wayne and I had settled on our plans for having all our time for ourselves. All his children and all my boys were on their own.

This was a frightening experience I faced-three little ones to care for completely. A two-month-old baby, a little girl of two years with leukemia, and a young man of four very emotionally unsettled by all that was going on around him. It was very difficult. Adjustments had to be made by all of us. Children, and adults alike. We all had our ups and downs, but we did not give up. God carried us through it all. We would never have made it otherwise.

Our first order of business was a visit to Crystal's doctor. I was more apprehensive about caring for her than I was about the other two. After that visit, I was more confident that I could handle the situation. We also visited Brian and Amanda's doctors so that we could also know exactly where we stood on care for them.

Our second order of business was plans for Christmas. It was the middle of December, and that the jolly old man in the red suit was expected by two little ones. The baby was too small to know, but Brian and Crystal fully expected that Santa not over look them. They were not so sure that he would find them since they had moved and it was such a short time till the big day. I assured them that Santa had a special way of keeping up with all the children, even ones that moved suddenly, and that he sure would not disappoint them.

Christmas morning came. Yes, Santa found just he right place to leave just enough toys to make eyes wide and hearts happy! It took lots of the Lord's blessings and a lot of legwork on my part (fast shopping that is), but we surely pulled it off in fine style.

I have said how frightening and difficult this period of time was, but praise the Lord, there were so many good and happy times too. I will forever be grateful to Him for giving me this time with the babies and for using me as their temporary haven.

I had a job as a grocery cashier. We needed what little money I earned, so I could not quit in order to stay home with the babies.

Everyone of my "family" at work went more than the distance to help me during this time. The ones who had baby furniture stored away, pulled it out and brought it to me to make my home life and work easier. They covered my work schedule for me many times with never a qualm. I was so very blessed to know and work with such caring God sent people.

The Lord led me to just the right person for babysitting duties at times that I had to be at work. Crystal's doctor would not approve of her attending a nursery. Her immunities were very low and even a bad cold could be bad news. Debbie had two children. A boy that was Brian's age, and a little girl that was Crystal's age. The little girl had low immunities like Crystal, as she suffered from kidney disease. The children all hit it off just fine and our little ones fell in love with Debbie. Debbie surely felt the same. She really enjoyed, also, having a little baby in the house again.

Our beautiful little Crystal lost her lovely golden hair as a side effect of the chemotherapy. She gained back her strength and weight and her zest for life, so we were very well pleased.

There were chemotherapy treatments every three weeks. In addition, every ninth week, there were two injections a day for five days. She took an antibiotic liquid twice a day because of the low immunities. She took three pills a day for five days after each chemotherapy treatment. There were lots of details and lots of big words that I could not quote to you if I had too. I did not even ask for a lot of them. I knew the doctor knew and that was what was important. I knew he was the best in the field of leukemia in children. I was confident in his ability and his desire to do all that could be done for our precious one. I knew that he had fallen in love with Crystal and wanted so badly for her to be one of his saves.

On one of our visits, he came into the room and said, "Well, how is our gal doing?" I answered, "She has been climbing up on the back of my couch trying to take the pictures off the wall!" His eyes lit up and he smiled as he replied with excitement, "That is wonderful!" I think it probably flashed through his mind as it did mine; that first day he saw her and how she looked as though she would never again have strength enough for such a feat.

The weeks turned into months as we pressed on regardless of anything. We made every trip to the doctor and the hospital that was needed. We took every pill and every spoonful of medicine that was prescribed. If not for those trips and medicines and that beautiful little bald head; we all but forgot about leukemia.

A picture I will always carry in my mind is one of the four of us on those steps at the doctor's office. Myself, and with Crystal in arm and Amanda in the other, and little Brian tagging behind. He was "Mema's helper;" because he would always run quickly past me up the steps so he could open the door for me.

July of 1982 rolled around, and it was time for the joint celebration of birthdays. Brian would be five this year and Crystal would be three. We held a nice party at our home and almost all the family members attended and had a very nice time.

Shortly after the birthday celebrations, Brenda decided that she had improved enough to be able to take the children to live with her. She had found a job and a small apartment and also felt capable of caring for them. Wayne and I had grown so close to them and so used to the confusion that we could not bear for them to be gone all the time. So there were times that I would go by the babysitters and pick them up and take them home with me just as I had been used to doing over the past several months.

We loved all three of them with all our hearts, but Amanda seemed like our very own baby. Nighttime feedings and changing, progression from formula to milk to baby food, watching as she learned to coo and turn over, finding that first tooth as it clinked against the spoon at feeding time...how could we have felt any different? I believe her instincts drew her closer to us, also. Crystal always had lots of love to give, but Mommy was the number one in her life; there was never any doubt about that. Amanda always seemed to be better satisfied with us,

Crystal with Mommy. As a matter of fact, Crystal was just a little jealous of attention Amanda got from Mommy, even though she lover her baby sister. Brian was "community property." He was fine wherever he happens to be and made the best he could out of all of it. Just as long as there was lots of running room, he was in good shape.

September came and Brian started kindergarten at school. Then Christmas seemed to come ever so fast. Michael and Brenda decided with us that the best place for the children for Christmas was at our home. I am so glad we did not miss this special time with them.

February 1983 came and brought great heartache and disappointment. Crystal relapsed and had to return to the hospital. It was as much a shock as it was the first time. We all refused to believe anything except that she would be cured. She looked so vital and healthy that we just could not believe otherwise. Now we had to give up a lot of our optimistic outlook because the doctor was telling us that if the first remission did not last for five years, and that the patient did not usually make it.

Remission came quickly this time. It was a possibility that there would be more remissions to be achieved, but each one would be shorter. We still held to our thread of hope.

Brenda quit work in order to spend all her time with and for Crystal. I spent more of the time I had away from work with Brian and Amanda. Not that I excluded Crystal, but she needed and desired her mommy "twenty-five" hours a day. She spent lots of time with her brother and sister too because she loved them dearly.

One evening Brenda called Brian and Crystal in from a time of play outside with the neighborhood children. Baths were necessary and Crystal decided to be the first. She stepped into the tub and sat down for mommy to bathe her. They always talked while this process was going on. Today, Crystal had been told something by one of her playmates that would have to be discussed with Mommy.

She looked up at her Mommy and asked a question that should have held no part of thinking for a child of three. "Mommy, one of my friends said I was going to die. Am I going to die Mommy?"

Now Brenda was experiencing one of those fleeting moments that seemed to last a million years. She choked back the tears and frantically scanned the passage of her mind for an answer. An answer that would be acceptable and comforting to such a small child, with surely such a lack of comprehension to whatever the answer would be. An answer to allay fears about this thing she had been "called to do" by an older and surely more knowledgeable person than herself. I will always believe that our gracious Lord stepped in and gave Brenda the words to speak, and she never realized what she said until she had time later to think it over.

She said, "Crystal, we all are going to die someday." This did not bring satisfaction for there was a second question.

"What happens when you die, Mommy?"

" You go to heaven to live with Jesus." was the answer.

"Where is heaven, Mommy?"

"It is up in the sky where the clouds and birds are." was her reply.

By this time, Brian had heard bits and pieces of this conversation and his curiosity would have to be satisfied, to, so he chimed in by asking, "What is heaven like, Mom?"

Brenda proceeded to explain. "It is a lovely place. Everything is beautiful. Jesus and God live there. Everybody is happy and nobody is sick. Everybody loves each other. The animals are all gentle and you can pet them. It is a very nice place."

This seemed to Brian the very place to be! What he remarked next turned what could have been a sad recollection into a pleasant memory. "That sounds neat, Mom! Can we pack our bags and all go there now together?"

"No," Brenda answered. "Each one of us has to wait for our own special call from Jesus."

This finally gained satisfaction and approval from both children, so that time went on as usual except for Brenda fighting back the tears.

Amanda was walking and talking by now, and she provided constant entertainment and pleasure for her older sister. Crystal especially loved to comb and fix her little sisters hair, not having enough of her own to notice. Remarkably, however hers had started to grow and to stay. It never came out again.

Amanda was very smart for her age and she retained almost all Crystal taught her. Their favorite game was:

"Ring around the roses,

Pocketful of posies,

Ashes, ashes, all fall down!"

The laughter rang through the house like tinkling bells when they played.

It was about this time that I received another "slight insight." I went by to visit the children after work one afternoon. Crystal had been playing at a neighbor's and was walking toward me as she came home. There was something different about her that I could not put clear substance too. As I kept watching her, puzzling about it, a thought flashed across my mind, "Get ready to let her go soon."

I believe our Lord also gave these insights to Crystal. One day while she and Brenda were in the yard, she called her Mommy's attention to some birds flying over head. "See those birds up there, Mommy." "I am going to go up there where they are soon."

As time raced on toward July and August and the usual joint birthday celebration, we wondered together just how to handle the situation. We decided that we had best have as special a time as we could. Though we tried to confine the thought to the deepest darkest parts of our hears and minds, we knew it would be the last one for our Sissy.

Party time came and Crystal looked radiant that day. She soaked up every moment of the special day. She knew, too, that it would be the last. Even though she didn't understand totally, she knew. We were to be shown in the remainder of her days, just how much more she did know than we did. More than she could share with us because it was special, just between her and Jesus.

Remission ended again.

It puzzled us when the doctor asked "if" we wanted to try for another remission. We just could not accept the lack of hope. We just did not fully understand that further treatments could cure, only prolong the inevitable. We heard correctly, as the doctor related all this to us, but it is strange that we still even now expected a miracle.

So, it was back to the hospital and more needles. Oh, how she hated those needles. The doctor and the nurses always said that she was the best they had ever known about tolerating those things that she hated most—the hospitals and the needles. She never struggled or tried to pull away. She always forgave and gave an "I love you" to them after treatments. She never blamed them for what they had to do to her.

I believe she knew that it was all so unnecessary now. She begged for no more—no more shots, and no more hospital. But we proceeded with a weekly trip to the hospital for an overnight stay for intravenous medicines, and a weekly trip to the doctor's office for blood count and checkup.

There was a task that preyed on my mind to be done. If our baby was to go back home to Jesus, I wanted her to look beautiful on her journey. This was a task that I thought I had better attend to in case time was shorter than expected. I had a picture in my mind of the way I wanted her to look, and it had to be a dress that I made for her. She always loved things the "Mema" sewed for her. So I went to the store and found some lovely pink cotton for a dress and white eyelet for an apron. It was looking for thread to match and came to a rack holding appliques for decorating children's clothes. One of them "jumped" out at me from its place on the rack. A little pink word with white wings on each side. "Angel"

I made the dress and was very pleased with the way it turned out. I did not mention it to Brenda, since she was in such stress already. She knew many details had to be attended to, but her strength failed at the very thought of them. I told her to just concentrate on Crystal's care, and I would attend to all else and everything would fall into place, as it should.

As the days progressed, we began to understand more fully why the doctor had asked "if" we wanted to proceed with more treatments. The next remission we prayed for was not to come. She begged more intently every day. "No more shots, please. No more hospital, please." So because of her pleas and the confirmation from the doctor that the remission would not come, Mommy and Crystal sat down to have a talk. It must have been the most heartbreaking conversation Brenda will ever have with anyone.

"Crystal, you have been asking for no more shots and no more hospital. Do you know what it means if we stop all that?"

"What, Mommy?"

"It means that you will have to go live with Jesus."

"That is what I want to do, o.k. Will you come with me, too, Mommy?"

The overpowering strength of God must have poured into Brenda to get her through this time as gracefully as she did.

"No, honey, I can't come with you now. I will have to stay here and wait till Jesus calls me. I can promise you that you will be very happy with Him and you won't be sick any more. Someday when He calls me we will be together again."

"O.K., I want you to let me tell the doctor myself about this when we go to see him."

She was promised that she could.

Even though she had made her decision, we were not sure that we could carry through with it. Brenda's sister called in the Pastor of her church to consult with us and lead us in the decision making prayer. We decided that Crystal knew best and we should uphold her in her decision.

That next trip to the doctor's office there were so many emotional extremes engrossing each of us. Crystal sat straight and tall and smiled at the doctor as he came into the room.

"Guess what?" I'm not going to have any more shots and I'm going to stay home and not go to the hospital any more!" Now the doctor smiled too, like the rest of us; through big tears welling up in his eyes and choking knots in his throat. His heart was breaking like ours to have to give in.

We decided that Michael and I should move into Brenda's apartment for the remainder of Crystal's days. She needed all those near that loved her, and all that loved her needed to help her through these last days. I took leave from work to be with my family.

I don't remember when exactly the next "slight insight" came. It was a feeling about a birthday and about the nighttime. My birthday was coming in September and so was Brenda's. This year we surely did not look forward to them.

I went ahead with arrangements that needed to be made. Crystal was pre-registered for death with the coroner's office. This is necessary for terminal patients who will die at home. It avoids much confusion, and we need to avoid all we could. I also went ahead with funeral arrangements so as to make it easier later on.

God had been very gracious to our little one as He carried her through this disease. Suffering had really been minimal in comparison to many cases. We gave Him praise for that as we beseeched His hand in carrying her the rest of the way. There were possibilities of horrible experiences such as convulsions, vomiting up blood and extreme pain facing such a wonderful little one. We dreaded the thought of what we might have to witness, but we mostly dreaded Crystal having to suffer. We prayed constantly that God in His graciousness would not let her suffer long and hard.

And gracious He was, too. He soon gave us evidence that Jesus was there. Crystal was resting in the bedroom on hers and Mommy's bed. Brenda was sitting on the bed at Crystal's feet. They had been chatting away but suddenly Crystal became very still and quiet. Her eyes seemed to set, staring at the ceiling. It frightened Brenda so badly that she grabbed the baby's feet and shook her and called her name loudly.

Crystal turned to look at her, peacefully but with questioning eyes. Brenda picked her up and came into the living room where I was sitting. She began to tell me what had happened and how it had frightened her so badly. It was then put aside until a short time later when Crystal brought it up. "Mommy, I saw someone in the bedroom a while ago. It was Jesus. He was on the ceiling over our bed." Now we knew for sure He was there to comfort her and He had allowed her to let us know so that we could share in this comfort.

There was a time I am sure I witnessed this communing with Jesus. She was lying on the couch and she became as Brenda had described before, very still and peaceful with eyes set on the ceiling. We did not bother her or ask her about it. We knew if she and Jesus wanted us to know, she would tell us.

One day during a chatting time, we were taken aback by a request made Crystal. She wanted to have Christmas! She was promised that soon, we would. We started plans for our September Christmas and the news, of it spread like wildfire. Everyone wanted to help, to participate, to be included in even the smallest way as a part of this celebration. Contributions of money came form many directions. Food and cakes were pledged for the big day. A close family friend brought a tree and we set it up and put all the decorations on it. Immediately, presents began to gather under that tree. A local photographer promised to come and take lots of pictures. The Shriners pledged clowns to liven up the party.

The big day came, but sadly, it was not one of Crystal's good days. The process of withdrawal from all the drugs had caused bad sores in and around her mouth. They were very painful, especially with she tried to talk or smile. It was also one of her weak days. But she still did her best to enjoy all of what was happening. She and Mommy decided that she could let us know when she was smiling by blinking her eyes. We had dressed her in a gown, thinking that she would be more comfortable. When Amanda enters all decked out in a pretty party dress, Crystal felt very underdressed. This brought on a change of clothes, of course, and then she was well pleased to be all prettied up. She had always been very meticulous with appearance.

She loved opening presents; so she made sure to conserve enough energy to gets that done. Her favorite gift was a Barbie doll from Mommy. That Mommy! She always knew just the right thing to get!

Everyone wanted to hold her and touch her. It was though each one felt they could inject some of their strength into her with a touch. They were all so concerned and well meaning. They just didn't know how it hurt her to be touched. She did desire closeness at times, though. She had learned that Mommy or Mema knew just how to hold her so that it didn't hurt quite so bad. She was usually very specific about what she needed and who she wanted to fulfill that need. That was what we were there for so we did the utmost we could to grant even the smallest request.

It was surely a very lovely Christmas. We were all tired when it ended. We were also filled to the brim with love and concern and compassion shown by so many friends and neighbors and family members.

Now we were through mine and Brenda's birthdays and Christmas. She began to have more days that she was not so weak. A period that the doctor called "false hope."

She took one of those days and crammed all she could into it. Brian asked her if he could kiss her and having been told yes, he kissed her lightly on the side of her mouth. As he pulled back from her, the scab fell from that ugly sore on her mouth. They both noticed it at the same time and broke into screams of laughter. "Mommy! Mema! My big brother kissed away my sore from my mouth." That was surely the high point of the day. She took time to stand in a chair at the sink and help me wash dishes. She went in the back yard with Daddy for some swinging on the swing set. She went with Mommy for a visit to Grandmother's house. They also made a stop to get fried chicken and mashed potatoes. She enticed Brian to sit in the high chair and put the tray on so that he could not get out. Then she proceeded to mark all over him with various colors of magic markers. When she let him get down and get in the tub, she laughed at his efforts to wash all those colors off. He did it, but it really took some scrubbing. Brian laughed just as hard over the whole ordeal as she did. He was in tune with the rest of us, to do anything to make her happy. As the day was drawing to a close, she put the last of her strength into going for a walk, with her in the stroller with Mommy.

One of the nurses had told us that playing of religious music and hymns had been found to be very soothing to terminal patients. Brenda had a record player that had been very spasmodic in its performance, but we gathered some records from friends and relatives and prayed for it to perform properly. It did! It never missed a lick of its duty, night and day, and it played on and on.

We took turns spelling, one another carrying or rocking her, as she would let us. She could not be let to walk alone. Her knees were just too wobbly. It happened to be my turn one evening. We sat in the rocking chair in the bedroom. We played the music box and admired all her pretty presents on the shelf by the bed. We especially enjoyed a lovely picture of Jesus and a beautiful little blonde girl that He held in His arms. This evening was a weak time, so as I talked to her, she just nodded her head from time to time, but did not participate in the conversation.

"Crystal, Jesus is surely a handsome man, isn't He? You can just tell how much He loves that little girl by the way He smiles and looks at her. She looks very happy too, because He is holding her, doesn't she? It looks, as though He is probably a tall man, doesn't it? I guess that little girl had to put her arms up to Him so He could take hold of her to pick her up, don't you? That is what you will have to do, too. When He reaches down for you, put your arms up to Him so it will be easier for Him to pick you up okay?" She nodded a slight yes and soon fell asleep. Even though she was asleep and no longer needed rocking, I sat holding her, trying to hoard a lifetime of closeness to her in my body, heart, soul and mind.

She told us twice more of Jesus' presence. Once He was lying on the bed beside her. The last time He was by her shoulder as she sat on the couch.

The doctor prescribed a strong painkiller called "Brompton's cocktail," as the time for the worsening of the pain approached. That is a mixture of cocaine, morphine and alcohol. The dosage when we started was one teaspoon every four hours. As time progressed the dosage became larger and the time between doses got shorter. It surely saved Crystal much suffering. At first, she would put off taking it as long as she could but she soon realized the ease it gave, and just, knew the right time to ask for it. She was such a brave little girl carrying such a big cross. She seldom cried or complained.

Even though she knew we were keeping our promise of no more shots, now she even dreaded the ride to the doctor's office. We went on Monday and Thursday. Her only conciliation was a stop on the way home to get fried chicken and mashed potatoes.

Monday, October 3rd, was a time for he doctor's office again. She really did not feel good today. She seemed to dread the trip more than she usually did, and even cried a little at having to go. During the visit, the doctor didn't do much or say much. I guess that was appropriate for there was nothing left to do or say. Crystal told him good-bye and gave him a weak kiss on the cheek. One could have sliced the emotion in that room with knife; it was just that thick.

Brenda asked him if he thought we would make it back for the Thursday visit. His reply was "We'll see."

As we were leaving the office I stopped by the front desk to speak to one of the nurses. She remarked that Crystal looked very low and would probably not last out the week. She also said, " Our fondest wish is that we could make well all who come to us, but when our medicines no longer work, that means Jesus is calling and there is nothing we can do about that."

We stopped for our prize of chicken on the way home. Crystal made me promise that I would go bring her Daddy home from work right away. After I got her and Mommy settled, it only took about half an hour to go get Michael and get back to the apartment. The scene that met us was not a pleasant one. Crystal had started vomiting large clots of blood. All that afternoon we suffered with our precious one, and prayed constantly for God's grace. And gracious He was. Miraculously it stopped after a few hours. The worst part of the whole ordeal for Crystal was the worry that she had ruined Mommy's blouse because she got blood on it. Even as desperately ill as she was, this was her main concern. Brenda assured her it would come out, but she was not satisfied until it was taken and washed so she could see proof.

She was able to rest most of the night, waking occasionally for water or her medicine. The nights had not really been too bad, but this night, we all hung on every breath she took.

Tuesday, October 4, she had made it through one more night. We were afraid she would have to suffer more vomiting, but the Lord spared her from that. There was only a trickle or two from her nose. She would not eat, only take small amounts of liquid. Her heart was strong, beating at 155 beats per minute for the last few days. She tried hard to stay awake.

That evening, the pastor came to help console us in what we now know now are her last hours. A nurse came to keep track of her vital signs and to confirm the time of death. At about 6 p.m., Crystal slipped into a coma. Her breathing was very labored.

At about 11 p.m., I was sitting in the living room with my oldest son, Doug. As a flash of memory came across my mind, it scared me so much that it took my breath away. Doug was concerned for me as he took my hand and asked if I was all right. I said, "Yes, I am all right. I just had a thought. If she goes after midnight, it will be Amanda's birthday!"

A short time later, Michael came into the room and said, "Mother, it will be soon now so you had better come hold her for a few minutes."

I went to the bedroom. She way lying on the bed. She looked peaceful except for the struggle to get air. It was to be her lungs that gave out first. I wanted more than anything to hold her, but the fear that

I would awaken her to suffer pain kept me from picking her up. I just sat down on the floor by the bed and held her All her family circled around her. Our pastor lead us in prayer for God's divine will to be done and to acknowledge His graciousness already bestowed. I could only pray that she would quietly slip away to Jesus with no more suffering. Brenda kept murmuring, "Go to Jesus, Sissy. Just go to Jesus, now. We all love you so much, but Jesus is the only one who can help you now."

At 12:42 a.m., October 5, she opened her eyes. They were clear and bright as she turned her head on the pillow and gave each one of us a short look. As her eyes met mine I felt her say "Bye, Bye, Mema". She turned from me and as she looked straight up she lifted her left arm and came up slightly off the bed, but fell back. She then raised both arms up as high as she could reach. They fell back to the bed, her eyes closed, and she was smiling. Jesus had picked her up.

Sorrow, relief, everything hit at once like a ton of bricks. Tears for the sorrow and laughter, for the joy of so vividly witnessing her going to His arms. I could only say "Praise God!" What infinite mercy and comfort He had showered on us.

After a prayer for continuing support from Him and praise for his mercy, Crystal was made ready for her trip to the funeral home. The nurse bathed her and rubbed her with lotion and put a clean gown on her. Each of us spent the last few moments holding and hugging her and whispering good-bye to her. I was asked later how I could have done such a thing. Only reply, "How could I not have done so? It was my last chance to hold her here on earth!"

She was taken away at about 3 a.m. We all decided we must try to rest, because the next two days would not be easy. The record player was turned off and we fitfully grabbed a short rest.

The next morning we arose to go to see our little girl all dressed up to go away. She was beautiful.

We returned home and the silence was so loud that we decided to turn the record player on again. We felt it would comfort us, as it had

Crystal. The switch was pushed on, but that record player would not start. It has never played again.

It has been almost a year now. Brenda found another job and I retired from mine. I wanted to care for Brian and Amanda while she worked.

There will always be a big empty space in our lives, but I feel very special and honored that I am. the proud grandmother of a beautiful little girl that was too good for earth so she lives with Jesus.

He is still attentive to me and showers of blessings still come to me. One night, not too long ago, I was especially lonesome for Crystal. As I slipped into bed and said my prayer for the night, I injected a request for a dream of her so that I could feel that I had visited her.

I awoke very fulfilled that next morning. During the night, I had been with Crystal. I don't know where we were, but she was sitting on my lap and I teasingly kissed her on the neck. It must have tickled for she wiggled and laughed. We both laughed and laughed.

No, I haven't lost her just because I cannot touch her with my hands or see her with my eyes. All I have to do is ask Jesus and then I can touch her with my heart and see her in my dreams.

# Raphael, A Guardian, A Friend

By

James Fleagle

While attending, Slidell Vo Tech., in Slidell, Louisiana, I worked part time delivering furniture. After a few short days, James, a fellow furniture deliverer, and I became friends. One of the after work items we enjoyed doing was fishing.

One place we enjoyed fishing had a service road leading to it. The first half was black topped, while the second half was made up of oyster shells in the middle of a 60 degree left hand turn. In Louisiana, or a least that part of Louisiana, they used oyster shells instead of gravel.

One evening we agreed to go fishing; most of the time James rode with me. That evening he declined, opting to come later. After work I found myself going fishing. Once turning off the main road and on the service road with Rod Stewart blasting out of my guaranteed speakers to last a lifetime, I had visions of hauling in a record catch prior to James's arrival.

I was in the turn where the oyster shells started, when I noticed my car was skating on the shells as if on ice. I was not going an excessive speed. I was told later, the shells had just been graded that day, thus having a surface like ice. Once exiting the turn, I noticed I was heading for cattails, not knowing if it was semi-solid ground or if it was swamp water. That area was swamp, as is most of Louisiana in that area. I didn't want to take any chances and steered to my left in the direction of a thirty-foot wide canal (creek for u northerners). The front of the car never changed directions, and stayed pointed straight sown. So not wanting to get wet I steered right. This time I was heading toward a telephone pole, and I knew for a fact, I did not want to run into it. I jerked the steering wheel to the left. That is when the front of the car changed directions and headed straight for the water. Not wanting to receive a neck injury, I lay down on the front seat and took the biggest breath I had ever taken in my entire life. The car came to rest upside down under water.

The car ran off the road and started going down the bank of the canal. At the water's edge, the front bumper dug into the mud, sending the rear end in the air. Now, I am not the smartest person on God's green earth, but I realized that the top of the car was now on the bottom. Figuring this I knew I had to reach down to touch the headliner. So, reaching down I searched for the open window. I searched about fifteen times. I then, swam to the passenger's side of the car and began another search for an open window on that side of the car. The same luck I had on the driver's side followed me to the passenger side of the car. At that point, I just knew I had bought the farm.

As I was running out of air, I pondered whether or not to go ahead and breath in as much water at once, maybe to get it over quicker, or just let it take it's own course. After explaining to myself how dumb I was for getting myself into this situation, a familiar voice came to me, my guardian angel Raphael. Raphael told me to try the driver's side once more. Well, he knew what he was speaking about. I found that elusive open window on the first try.

Once pulling myself out of the car and sinking knee deep into sewage mud, I realized it was alligator mating season. During this time of the year the alligators get a bit testy about foreign objects in their waters. It didn't take a rocket scientist to tell me to get my hind-end out of there in short order.

Once the wrecker had pulled the car out of the water, I realized the top of the car had come to rest on a fallen tree trunk or a telephone pole, and the roof was shaped in a "V". This was the only reason the top of the car did not sink into the sewage mud.

This is another time I must have put another gray hair on Raphael's head. Without his intervention I would have become a gator entree for that evening.

I have been giving him thanks for that incident as well as many others for pulling my fat out of the fire. I think I am on the path I am to travel, healing and teaching. Through the wet times, as well as the dry, Raphael has been for and with me.

Thank you my Friend.

James Fleagle

# Introduction:
# Divine Healing

My walk with Jesus Christ, my Lord and Savior in the past 7 years of my heart disease, has been one of utmost love, joy, heartache and healing. We are flesh, in the physical sense, and placing our hope in the spiritual realm with our faith. When I was rushed to the hospital, literally dying, my spirit told me I was leaving this world. I cannot say that at that time I was fearful of dying, because my physical body was so very ill. After my long recovery, I began to ask questions of "Why?" Why did I survive this horrible heart attack only to live with constant disease in my body and fear of the unknown?

I began to search for the answer, only to realize that I was to know the answer when it was God's time for me to know.

God has given me my answer...A healing ministry of words on a printed page, a written dedication of my life to believing and sharing the miracles of the power of the cross. He has shown me so many signs and wonders of his power and presence since my illness. His presence is unmistakable in my life, because he has given me the ability to discern His voice and feel the hearts of people. I glorify my Heavenly Father in all that I do. Through prayer, I seek his face for the answers to all life's questions and trials. I know that God heals the sick of disease that invades the body and mind. Scripture is very clear on the subject of healing. For the three short years that Jesus ministered on Earth, He healed multitudes of people. Christian teaching tells us that

He died on the cross, not only for our salvation, but also for the healing power of His blood. It was all a part of God's divine plan for us. He died so that we might live for eternity and to also have whole and healthy bodies. In Isaiah 53:5, the scripture plainly reveals to us "He was wounded for our transgressions, He was bruised for our iniquities: the chastisement of our peace was upon Him; and with His stripes we are healed." God does not lie, and that fact you can depend on. Prayer, praise, faith and thanksgiving are the answers to our healing. We must accept that He lives in us. He shed his blood on the cross two thousand years ago so that healing and salvation was fulfilled as part of our inheritance in God's divine plan.. Accept this, thank him for it, and stand in faith that you are healed.

Dr. Michael De Vita's book reminds us that "When you pray to God, expect an answer. Be prepared for the answer that God has for you. His plan for you may be totally different from what you're asking for or what you expect. His ways are truly higher than ours, and His thoughts are truly higher than ours. He gives beyond what we can ask or even think. We need to be prepared for this when we pray."
Excerpt: From his book: The God of Abraham, Isaac, Jacob and me, by Michael DeVita, M.D.

"While it cannot be denied that the New Testament teaches that God did heal many people supernaturally in the first century. There are many in the church today that would be keen to downplay the present day relevance of such examples for those presently suffering with various forms of sickness and disease. The ministry of divine healing in the name of Jesus has been especially controversial in the last century, and has stirred up much religious feeling on both sides of the issue. At times this has been at least in part due to the unwise practices of certain well-known "faith-healers." In some cases people have rejected divine healing because they could not accept some of the doctrines and practices of those who advocated it. Yet the Scripture does speak on this issue, and it is of great relevance to those who are sick and suffering, if perchance Jesus Christ might still be willing to demonstrate his compassion and power by healing them.

Michael Frackerell (www. christian-faith.com)

We must be willing to "test all things," and "hold fast to that which is good." Our standard of reference for discerning truth must be the Scriptures themselves, and not the pronouncements of popes, reformers, theologians, pastors, teachers or evangelists—although all of these may have something worthwhile to say at times."

Pray for God's hand to touch you with HIS healing power, then claim this power in the name of Jesus. Believe that you received your healing and never doubt it. Regardless of the circumstances around you, never doubt God's ability to heal you. Give him praise and thanksgiving for your blessings. Psalm 100:4-5 tells how to approach our Heavenly Father. "Enter into his gates with thanksgiving, and into his courts with praise, be thankful unto him, and bless his name. For the Lord is good; his mercy is everlasting; and his truth lasts in all generations." Surrender your life to Him, and He will direct your path and be the Lord of your life.

The Holy Spirit spoke to me personally while in prayer early one morning. It was so beautiful and so quiet. His still soft voice was comforting and clear. He said to me, "I am the Lord thy God that healeth thee." Those beautiful words are an everlasting reminder to me that Jesus Christ is truly the author of my faith and the Lord of my Life.

The assurance that I am never alone in my life fulfills all my needs. I to truly know that he will never forsake me or leave me. His Grace has proven to be truly sufficient.

*"Bless the Lord, O my soul, and forget not all His benefits: Who forgives all your iniquities, Who HEALS ALL YOUR DISEASES, Who crowns you with loving kindness and tender mercies, Who satisfies your mouth with good things, So that your youth is renewed like the eagle's."*
*Psalm 103:2-5*

# Healing Testimony
## by
## Brother Gordon Dacre

November, 1999

The testimonies are just to numerous too write at this time, however, the first of the heart miracles I encountered was in 1995. I was ministering in a meeting and the Lord spoke to me and said that there was one present that had a problem and that they were ready to receive their healing.

I called out the situation and a lady promptly stepped forward with her sick son. The son received immediate healing in his body. Before returning to her seat, the Lord showed me that the mother was also sick with a heart problem. She was so consumed with her son's problem, that she had forgotten her own need.

Two months after praying for her, I received a letter from the mother. Dear Brother Gordon,

The night you prayed for my son and I, you were not to know that I was suffering from an incurable heart problem. You prayed for me and laid your hands on me. At first I felt nothing, but as the days passed I began to get stronger. Eventually, I went for my monthly treatment at the University teaching hospital. The doctor examined me three times and then left the room only to return some time later with a team of student doctors. They all started running tests, and inquired what the problem was. I was then informed that not only was there no trace of the problem, but that I appeared to have a new heart altogether.

Since that time I have seen countless thousands of healing and miracles. The Lord spoke to me and said, teach my people how to receive their miracle, teach them how to keep their miracle, and then teach them how to become vessels for miracles.

That is why I was sent to this country.

Gordon

*"These signs will follow those who believe: In My Name, they will
lay hands on the sick and they shall recover."*
Mark 16:17,18

# Michael's Testimony

Let me begin by saying that it is a miracle I ever got saved. In the
gospels, Jesus reserved his hardest words for the Pharisees. He told them
prostitutes and tax collectors were entering the Kingdom of Heaven
first. Folks, in my heart I was at least as bad as the worst Pharisee.

My parents come from a Dutch Reformed (Calvinist) background.
I thank God for their Godly influence on me. Every night, they would
pray before meals and after the meals Dad would read a portion of the
Bible to us. I think we covered most of the Bible in this way. They put
into me the habit to go to church twice on Sundays, to respect certain
standards of morality and lots of good things. As I grew up I considered
myself to be a Christian. Why? I believed the Bible was the Word of
God, that Jesus died for me to pay for my sins and that I was doing
what other Christians did.

In the stream of Christianity in which I grew up, it was very
commonplace to do Bible studies. I was very proud of my ability to
know the stories and have an opinion on everything. I grew up with the
feeling that I had the right religion and that I was better than other
people. I was so proud of my academic results at school. I looked down
on others and had little regard for their feelings. As a result, I failed to
develop socially.

As I entered into adolescence, I had a hyperactive mind. It was
constantly thinking and planning according to the thought "What's in it
for me?" It was constantly seeking to inform me of things to feed my

pride. My grandmother said to me a few years ago, "Michael, when you were growing up, you were a ball of pride."

At the same time I was convinced that I was a Christian. I knew I had sins and was basically selfish, but I had confidence that I was saved because I mentally assented to the doctrine of the substitutionary atonement of Christ. There were times, however, when certain people made me uneasy, because of their obvious joy in serving the Lord and their clear proclamation that they were no longer their own masters, and that they were living for Jesus and not for themselves. During such times, I was always waiting for an escape so I could get back to enjoying my various hobbies and avaricious pursuits.

I went to the University with the determination to be a great computer scientist. I guess I was a computer nerd. I'd written my first commercial game program at fourteen in 1980 and I know now that the love of computers (which were essentially tools to praise my cleverness and me) was a major form of idolatry in my life. But I was sure I was a Christian! I had felt sorry about some of my sins and had even asked Jesus into my heart! I was doing what others in church were doing! I could discuss theology with the best of them! I was outwardly moral, principled etc., but utterly self-centered.

The one thing I was most uncomfortable with in those days was witnessing. Being socially backwards and with more than my share of acne on my face, it was not something I wanted to do, especially with strangers.

But there came a day when a young ethnic Chinese man from Campus Crusade for Christ gave me a call on the phone and invited me to meet with him. I don't know why I agreed, but I did. Over the next few months with this man, my life began to change. He helped me to start telling the gospel to others. Doesn't the Scripture say that if we keep on confessing Christ as Lord and believe God raised Him from the dead, we will be saved? Strange as it may seem, it was at this point that I believe I truly surrendered my heart to God. For I had surrendered to Christ the thing I was most unwilling to do for God. And I think until we come to that point, we still have not received Christ as Lord. Until that point, we do not really belong to Christ. I didn't know that Jesus had to be Lord before His saving work on the cross was applied to your life.

That act of obedience on which surrender to Christ could be different for different people. For some, it could be in fact baptism in water. For another person, it might be commitment to a local church. For another, it could be simply a willingness to call upon the name of Jesus. What is important is that we yield to Christ on the point where our old nature wants to resist the most, for whatever reason. Then we are on the path of true faith. Mental assent is not enough. After the heart is surrendered to Christ, we will eventually be changed in every area in which we hear the Word of God rightly divided and act in faith on that.

One of the surprising things for me was the joy I found that in doing the thing I was most fearful of…to talk with others about Christ. What I found was that Christ became real to me as I went in His name. Before that, I knew lots of Bible and had done some things for God, or so I thought. But I was miserable. However, taking these first steps in living for God released a joy and happiness in me that I was not expecting.

Some of you may be asking, "But when were you baptized in water?" Well, that came later. You see, it is not baptism in water that justifies us. The important thing is that one submits His life to the Lord Jesus Christ. That way, the free gift of pardon and peace with God obtained at the cross can be ours. There is no way to be at peace with God if you are inwardly rebelling against his desire to govern your life. The only way to be in the Kingdom of Heaven is for Jesus to be your King! You can get baptized in water by the greatest saint in the greatest church without truly surrendering your heart to God. However, once you do surrender your heart to God, then if by God's grace you can get past all the theological murkiness that has historically covered the issue of baptism, and you understand that it is God's will for you. You will want to get baptized. This is what happened to me.

But there were still other things that the Lord did before He could get me to that point.

This is part II of my personal testimony. I share it hoping that it will bring glory to God and maybe even help someone else come to know the Lord better!

Many people have amazing dramatic testimonies. Its true—some people get off drugs miraculously and become the most radiant, wonderful joyful people so quickly that you can wonder: "God, what about the rest of us?"

I believe that salvation is both a package and a process. Our sanctification through faith in Christ is a process, although it can certainly have some powerful life changing events in the midst of it.

At the time when I started living for God, back in 1984, there were still a lot of things that God wanted to deal with in me. (I'm sure there still are!) Until that time, my desires had been after intellectual stimulation and personal recognition based on performance. I was still into computers pretty heavily and still played Dungeons and Dragons with my friends at times, sometimes until the early hours of the morning. I was no longer playing in a rock and roll band as I had done in high school, but I was still listening a lot to the radio.

It still seemed to me in many ways that the really appealing things were in the realm of fantasy, and that reality was kind of boring. Yet, God had begun to work in my life. The fact that my pursuits did not always coincide with my belief in the gospel didn't worry me too much, since most of the other Christians I had ever seen were the same.

Late in 1984, while in my second year in the University, I came across some people who talked about a dimension of spiritual life to which I had to admit I was a stranger. I wasn't sure if it was real. Around the same time, the popular Anglican [Americans read Episcopalian] preacher we listened to began to preach about the Holy Spirit. I didn't realize it at the time, but he was preaching against charismatics. The effect his preaching had on me, however, was to stir up curiosity. We had been so well taught that the Bible was the final authority on matters of faith, so I decided to check things out against the Bible. I was not satisfied with this preacher's response to my question: "If being filled with the Holy Spirit in the New Testament meant one thing—why doesn't it mean that anymore?"

Anyway, these people (who turned out to be charismatics), invited me to one of their small groups. I decided to check it out. I remember feeling really out of place there. Everyone had their hands in the air and the leader was saying, "Come on. Just reach out and touch God!" I thought it was silly to think of God being in the ceiling somehow.

I wasn't particularly impressed with what I saw. I thought; that the so-called prophecies, anyone could have made them up. But then again, who knows? Maybe there is something in it. I asked a lot of questions. I said, "If you guys are right, where are the miracles?" The leader said words to the effect of "We're getting there."

The leader of that group came and visited me in my college dorm, wanting to pray with me, but I put him off, since the exams were near.

Two other things happened around that time. One was, my mother gave me a tape from a charismatic Anglican preacher about the Holy Spirit and speaking in tongues. It turned out my mother spoke in tongues, but she had not wanted to push it on me. The other thing was my best friend told me he had started to speak in tongues while he was alone in his room.

Another event worth mentioning is that God led me to ask forgiveness from my father for certain things and to forgive him myself. I believe this was very important for what was to come.

I continued my search, reading the passages in the New Testament and wanting to know more. I visited an Assembly's of God church with my friend. I was under the impression that Pentecostals were like a cult...pretty heretical. Imagine my surprise when I heard the preacher preaching Jesus Christ and Him crucified, and salvation through the blood of Jesus. I concluded it couldn't be that bad after all. I'm so glad it wasn't some fund raising message or something really far out that day, like you can find from time to time in Pentecostal churches.

I ended up seeking this pastor out at his house, without invitation. After sharing with me, we arranged another appointment. What really impressed me about this pastor was that he had seen blind eyes open in Jesus' name. God had also saved his life miraculously in an amazing way. I sensed he was telling the truth.

On the second appointment, he asked me, "Do you believe you will speak in tongues when I pray for you?" I said I wasn't sure, but he assured me it would happen. I was scared that nothing would happen.

To cut a long story short, I prayed to the Lord something like this: "Dear Lord Jesus, I want you, and only you. Fill me with the Holy Spirit and give me the power of God." I prayed this prayer based on Luke 11:13. God will give his children the Holy Spirit if they ask not a serpent.

I believed that I should open my mouth and speak what came out— so I did. At that very instant something very surprising happened to me. I felt like 240 Volts of power was going through my body—it was also a bit like pins and needles. I thought, "Something real is happening." I had never experienced anything like that before. At the same time, I continued to utter syllables that I did not comprehend at all. It was something that was right outside my experience. I had never felt anything like that when I prayed before! I knew it was God's power that I had asked for.

I went home and kept praying in tongues. Then I went to a Christian conference organized by Campus Crusade. I noticed in my life a greater desire to serve God, a desire after holiness and purity, which I had never known before. Up until that time, holiness had a very negative connotation for me…something like doing the dishes. But now things were different. The first unbeliever I talked with prayed to receive Christ.

When I returned to University, I knew that what I had experienced was not going to be accepted by most of my Christian friends. And I was right. I had already made the commitment though, that I was after truth no matter what it would cost me in terms of social relationships. I have never regretted that decision.

I started attending an AOG church. It wasn't long before the matter of water baptism was brought up. Having now experienced the Holy Spirit in a new way, I was eager for everything God had for me. I had long suspected that baptism was for believers, not babies. I remember wishing I could be baptized before as a believer when I was in the Anglican Church. I was glad to learn that it was part of God's plan. Accordingly, I was baptized in water in July 1985. To me this was also an act of consecration. No longer was I to live for the old desires, for the old nature. I was dedicating myself "unto all righteousness."

In 1985, while in my final year of University studying computer science, several significant events took place in my life, which changed my life and destiny. I had gone to University with the plan to become a great computer scientist. I wanted to do honors in Sydney and then a Ph.D. at Stanford University in the States, and I was very much on track until the end of my third year at University. But these goals and ambitions seemed less and less meaningful to me after the encounter I had with the Holy Spirit.

This encounter with the Holy Spirit made an impact on my world-view. I had entered into a totally new realm about which I knew very little. Many of the assumptions which I had held about the way God works in the world and which parts of the New Testament were relevant to me, I had been forced to modify.

Many different things started to happen in my life in 1985. I had an increased desire to win souls to Christ. But more than that, I wanted to know why the Pentecostal church I belonged to fell so short of the mark as far as revealing the truth of the promises which I had previously assumed to be "not really for today."

Don't get me wrong. That church had a great record as far as evangelism and church planting, and in the twenty years in 1977 from when it was planted from nine adults and five children it has grown to a worldwide movement with tens of thousands of people involved. However, my soul was reaching out for something more.

Why was it, for example, that there was so much talk about divine healing and so little concrete evidence that it was actually happening? My mind rebelled also against the teaching that one should say that they were healed even when there was still no sign of change. The whole thing seemed unreal.

Meetings with loud contemporary music, enthusiastic preaching and salvation appeals that drew ten to fifteen new decisions for Christ every meeting, but where was the promised power of healing so much talked about?

Earlier that year, however, I had been to a meeting organized by a charismatic pastor who invited a certain old gentleman by the name of Gordon Gibbs to preach there. Oddly enough, it was my mother who took me along there. I was pretty skeptical still about divine healing even though I had spoken in tongues and knew that was real.

There were about a hundred people at this meeting. After the time of praise this old preacher was introduced. It was nothing like I expected. Basically, all he did was share different stories from his experiences with God, and a few texts of Scripture. He didn't shout—he just talked, and he had the funniest mannerisms.

What was interesting though was what was happening on the inside of me. This incredibly warm presence gripped me in the area of the stomach. I can't describe it exactly, but it was like molten iron was in my belly (but absolutely no pain). I found myself absolutely riveted by the presence of God in the place.

Then something equally astonishing took place. The preacher had finished preaching, and some had come forward for salvation. But the meeting didn't end there. The preacher started calling out all these medical and emotional conditions, not general ones like back problems that someone is bound to have but very specific things. It seemed like he called out about thirty different things and always it matched someone in the crowd exactly. People were coming forward, receiving prayer, falling to the crowd, and getting up testifying that the pain was gone.

At the time, I had RSI from typing too much at computer keyboards. He never called that condition out, but what I noticed was that the blood in my hands started circulating very quickly it seemed, and the pain left.

Some friends of mine and myself returned with an unsaved friend to another one of these meetings. It was much the same, but this time, the preacher started naming the problems that our friend had. Our friend would not respond. But the preacher kept going into things in more and more detail. When my friend still refused to come out the preacher addressed him personally in front of everyone and asked him to respond. He got saved that night, and is in the ministry today.

All this put in me a strong desire to know God like this preacher did. Yet in the church I was attending, it seemed there was more smoke than fire.

Another important thing happened to me in August 1985. One night I had a dream in which I saw what seemed to be the faces of a multitude in darkness being sucked down into everlasting perdition. I woke up so shaken by that dream. I said, "God, I want to be an evangelist. But I'm asking you to confirm this by giving me 5 prophetic words from others in the next ten days.

What was interesting was that although people didn't usually prophesy to me, in the next ten days I did receive five prophetic words, which indicated to me that I should make the preaching of the gospel my central activity. One of them was from a preacher. He said in the name of the Lord, "I've been calling you for a long time. And don't let a career get in the way." This was significant for me because in those days I had the opportunity to earn big bucks with my computer skills. I had made $10,000 at least in my third year of University without much effort and it seemed the world could offer me a lot in that area. But now my direction was to change. Money meant nothing to me, and winning souls meant everything.

Around this time, I was still agonizing about the Scriptures concerning divine healing (like Ex. 15:26; Ps. 103:3; Is. 53:4,5; Jas.

5:14; Mk 16:17,18; John 14:12;Matt. 8:16,17) and many others. I wanted to believe it was true, but I could not! I felt tortured in my mind whenever I considered the matter. I had already seen some concrete evidence for it in life, but the failures in this area were all too evident to me also.

Determined to obey God whatever the cost, I finished my University degree without doing my honors year, and I entered into student evangelism on the Universities.

http://www.christian-faith.com/truestories.html

God bless you,

Michael

*"Daughter, your Faith has made you well. Go in peace, and be healed of your affliction."*
*Mark 5:34*

# My Testimony and Miracle
By
Judy Rogers

A tragic accident occurred, a little girl not quite five years old, was being pulled out of the water and given mouth-to-mouth resuscitation. The mother, in a panic-stricken state of shock, suddenly realized that because of her own backsliding condition she had never told the little girl about Jesus.

The man who had been working on her looked up and said, "I'm sorry, I cannot get her to breathe." Her frail little body had already turned grayish in color. The mother fell on her knees and cried out to God. "Please Lord, let her live so I can tell her about you."

About that time, the ambulance drivers came. The look on their faces told her she had lost her little girl. In desperation, she cried out louder, "Lord, please let her live so I can tell her about you." A huge crowd had formed, and ordinarily the mother would be too embarrassed to say she had ever given her life to Jesus, but the crowd didn't seem to bother her now, and she continued to cry out to the Lord.

The ambulance drivers had seen many drowning cases and just shook their heads and said, "we're sorry, she's gone." Then a miracle took place. God breathed the very life back into the little girl. The ambulance quickly took her to the hospital. The mother listened to the doctor as he sadly told her, "She's still unconscious and in a coma. We'll have to keep her and watch her carefully, there could be brain damage."

The mother went into the hospital room and knelt by the little girl's bed. She talked to God again and said; "Even if she lives and there is brain damage, she won't understand when I tell her about Jesus." Then God opened the eyes of the little girl and she said, "Mommy, why are you crying?" Well, that mother never stopped telling the little girl about Jesus and today that little girl is all grown up and now she is telling others about Jesus.

I thank God that I'm able to tell you this story. I'm the mother and Trena is that little girl. With the music ministry God has given us, our goal is to draw families closer to God and each other.

Judy and Trena

*"Jesus took my sicknesses and carried my pains, and by his wounds I am healed." Isaiah 53:4,5*

# Debbie

This testimony of healing is from a friend (also named Debbie). It is an awesome testimony to the healing power of Jesus Christ! Praise the Name of Jesus for He alone is worthy of all praise!

I have been a Christian since I was nine years old. I have always lived for the Lord.

I have had a lot of trials and heartaches. In 1982, I had cancer in a class 4b stage.

I had Hodgkin's Disease. It had spread into my bone marrow. I was given six months to live, unless chemotherapy did a miracle. I was on chemotherapy for 10 months. I went past my six months, thank God. I went to a Spirit-filled revival and GOD healed me!

That morning, I had gone for my chemotherapy and x-rays and my doctor told me I was still in poor condition. That night, I could hardly walk and was so sick at my stomach from chemotherapy, but I wanted to go to this revival so bad…my mom took me. I was called out of the audience and was anointed with oil. I knew instantly that I had been healed cannot explain the feeling, but it was like nothing I have ever felt before, or have felt since then.

It was wonderful. I went in for chemotherapy the next morning and I told my doctor I did not want to take chemotherapy because the Lord had healed me. He told me he believed in miracles, but the test the day before showed him differently. I ask him to redo the tests. He said no. He explained to me that if I did not take the chemotherapy he would no longer be responsible for my health.

My mom begged me to take the chemotherapy for her, so I did. Within the next 45 minutes after chemotherapy, I was on my way home and I became deathly ill and had an instant high fever.

My mother took me back to my doctor. I was rushed to the emergency room and put in isolation for 9 days (no visitor's etc). My mom could stay, but she had to stay with me 24 hours a day because everything had to be sterile. She even had to wear hospital clothes. My doctor thought I had hepatitis, or something contagious.

Then, it was all kinds of other infections. Every time, the tests came back clear.

Finally after the ninth day he admitted that I no longer had cancer! I had seven different kinds of infections because my body had rejected the chemotherapy. Praise the Lord a million times! I have been in remission ever since!

When I was diagnosed with Multiple Sclerosis, I guess I was in shock. I could not believe that I could have another major illness, especially since God healed me from cancer. I still believe GOD can heal me, but if he chooses not to—that is okay too. Many people are not as fortunate as I have been to have a healing like I have had, and by all rights, I should be dead. But through God's grace I have lived fifteen more years that I would not have been blessed with. I am doing my best to live everyday to it's fullest and not worry about what could or could not happen with the MS I grew up in a very Christian home and was "saved" when I was twelve. I tried to live the life of a Christian until I graduated from high school, but it never seemed very real to me. Even after high school and I was married, and thoughts of religion kept creeping into my consciousness.

But you see, my problem was that I had never really met this Jesus that everyone always talked about—at least not as a real person—never the "relationship" that I always heard so many other people talk about.

Through the years I tried to fill that void with many other things (like my marriage, my children, my career, etc.). As fulfilled as I was with these things, I always knew there was something lacking.

I wanted to find God. I wanted to find Jesus, but having grown up in the church, there was nothing new anyone could tell me! I knew that Jesus died on the cross for me and forgave me of my sins and that someday I would die and go to heaven, but it all seemed so void of feelings.

At one point in my life, I had pretty much given up finding what so many other Christians seemed so happy to have. I threw out everything "Christian" in my house except for Bibles, because I knew that would be "wrong." I had given up all hope of having a "relationship" with Jesus because I just thought it was impossible. I thought, maybe all the other Christians were faking it or, maybe if it was true. I wasn't good enough to be able to have this relationship with Him.

Then several years later, I was facing major surgery. But still, I would not turn to Jesus. I had promised myself that I would never turn to Him just because I was afraid, or needed Him because I had seen too many people do that and then go back to their old lives afterwards.

I did go through the surgery, and I was very sick for quite a few days. I remember my brother, who is a pastor sitting beside my bedside praying and praying . Still, I would not call upon the name of Jesus!

It wasn't until several weeks later, and I had gone to one of my brother's services (from a promise that I had made to him to attend) that the question was asked, "If you died tonight, do you know where you would go?"

Wow, that really made me start to think! I had pushed the idea of heaven and hell out of my mind for so many years! So, I decided to seek this Jesus one more time at the altar.

You may not believe this, but, I found out that JESUS IS REAL! Hallelujah!

He came to me that night in a way that I never thought possible!

I knew for the first time, what all those other Christians are talking about! He filled me with a Love so great, that I couldn't contain it within myself. He began speaking to me and leading me like He was just right beside me (which of course, He was)!

About a year after I had rededicated my life back to Jesus, and I knew that the Lord was calling for an even deeper relationship. He wanted to give me more of His Spirit and provide me with more power to be able to live a more victorious life, and that is when I received the Baptism of the Holy Spirit.

There's no way that I could ever convince you that Jesus is real. All I have is what I know and have experienced. It has been over seven years since I gave my life back to the Lord and it is still as sweet as the first day! I write this only to encourage you to keep on seeking Him! It may seem like an impossible journey, but when you seek Him, you WILL find Him, when you seek Him with your whole heart! (Jer. 21:13)

The choice is yours.

Please remember to pray for Debbie as she deals with the Multiple Sclerosis, and waits her healing from the Lord!

*"For I will restore health unto thee, and I will heal thee of thy wounds, saith the Lord"*
*Jeremiah 30:17*

# Mary Crane, Her Testimony

Friday, August 27, 1999, was just another day, except for the exhaustion I felt. My son, Richard Joseph, had been sick in the middle of the night again. It seemed he was not yet over a flu bug. My husband stayed home with him so that I could spend the afternoon with my mom and daughter, Rebecca.

We decided to eat lunch at a restaurant on the eastside of Milwaukee, but at the last moment, we changed our minds and chose another restaurant. It happened to be across from a Milwaukee County library, so we thought we would make a quick stop there. On the way we encountered a gentleman who greeted us kindly. He happened to be a Christian minister who was standing on the street corner chatting with people.

Upon leaving the library, this gentleman began talking to us. Oddly, he informed us that someone in the family had a sinus infection. I could only think of my aunt has frequent sinus infections, so I simply dismissed his comment. Then he mentioned that Rebecca was musical and played the piano. Yes, he was correct, we politely smiled and kept walking, wondering why he was saying these things to us.

As my mother crossed the middle of the road, he called out to her that she had a back condition and placed both of his hands on the lower back in the buttock area. My mother turned around and her mouth dropped open. We stopped and looked at him, not knowing what to say. For my mother had had surgery in that exact area a week ago and was recovering from it. How did he know these things? He cried out, "I just want you to praise the Lord!"

We didn't know what to think of this minister, except that we had experienced his warmth and kindness. He was right on two of the three things, but not on the sinus infection.

When I arrived home I found that my son was still sick. This was the third day, and I wondered why he wasn't getting better. He had missed going fishing and now had missed his first soccer game.

I dreaded another night of being awakened and feeling helpless when Richard Joseph cried. I was already exhausted from a long day so I went to bed early and tried to sleep. But I simply could not forget that gentleman's words, "Someone in your family has a sinus infection." As I tossed in bed these words would not leave me.

I considered a sinus infection like a mild cold…not a very serious condition, yet I kept thinking about that man. I decided to get up and check out some medical books. What startled me was the fact that sinus infections can lead to fevers. Richard Joseph had been having terrible headaches, stomach nausea, and at times a fever hovering around 103 degrees.

I began to wonder could his prescription be causing this? The doctor had not mentioned any dangerous reactions and the pharmacy had not given us any printouts. I studied the insert, which listed possible reactions to this medication in very technical language. Richard Joseph's symptoms matched almost all of them! I quickly telephoned the doctor who was on call and asked him if this medication could cause sinus infections. To which he replied, "Yes, the symptoms are similar," and he advised us to take him off the prescription immediately. I felt chills go down my spine as I realized this minister had been right—again.

The next night when Richard Joseph wasn't given any medicine, he finally slept soundly with no fever or headache. Each day he regained his strength and is now hundred. Praise the Lord! Yes, from this experience I learned the importance of asking the doctor and pharmacist about possible side affects and possible dangerous reactions from any medication. I felt so stupid that I had missed this now so obvious connection.

However, I can't forget the minister's last words to us, "I just want you to praise the Lord!" God had used him to warn us and to protect Richard Joseph. Is all this mere coincidence or just due to our medical ignorance? I believe God stepped into our ordinary day to stop us in our tracks and say, "I know you and I care about you!" How often have I ignored God's presence and taken God's blessing and people in my life for granted? I can only thank God for this gift of grace, and sending a stranger our way to remind us to "Praise the Lord!"

*"And one of them struck the servant of the high priest, cutting off his right ear. But Jesus answered, "No more of this!" And he touched the man's ear and healed him." Luke 22:50-51*

# The Testimony of Taunya Dowell

My name is Taunya Dowell and I'm 31 years old. I would like to share my testimony with you on the Miraculous Power of my Lord Jesus Christ.

When I was eleven years old, I was playing football with some boys and I was tackled. As a result, I fractured my left hip. I went through three surgeries and was in a cast from the waist down for a year and a half. My hip did not heal as the doctors had expected and over the years my left leg did not grow normally, and it ended up being one inch shorter than the right. I had MRI's done that determined the discrepancy in the length of my legs. I had a 1 inch build-up was made for all my left shoes. I continued to suffer from constant pain until one day in June of 1996,when a miracle happened.

I met Hal, who shared with me his healing ministry. My faith in Jesus was strong and I believed in the Bible and what it said. And when he shared with me the miracles he had seen through the power of prayer and calling on the power of Jesus, I wanted this for myself, and believed it was possible.

It was a beautiful sunny day in Coronado, California. When I crawled out of bed that morning, I was totally unprepared for a miracle. What happened changed my life forever. But God works his wonders in mysterious ways. Hal and I were sitting outside at a restaurant when he asked me if I would like to receive prayer. I was a little shy at first since we were out in public but then I said, "Let's do it." So he sat across from me and took both my ankles in his hands, with my legs stretched out, and started praying and invoking the power of the Holy Spirit in the name of Jesus and commanded my leg to grow. My left leg started getting very hot right above my knee and my bone started growing. My bone grew a whole inch right before our very eyes. I was so filled with the awesome power of the Holy Spirit I could barely think straight. I was awe-struck for hours. I had to go barefoot because my shoes will not fit anymore. My doctor checked me and they are at a loss for words. It has been over two years and I still don't need to have a lift in my shoe. I give all the glory to Jesus and now I have also learned how to pray for others to be healed. Based on Mark 16: 17-18, I feel we are called to pray for others for healing. It is the power of the Holy Spirit that does the healing, not anyone else.. The Lord just needs laborers to deliver the blessing.

*"He healeth the broken in heart, and bindeth up their wounds."*
*Ps 147:3*

# HEALING TESTIMONY
## By
## BILL HITT

I was in the Methodist church since before I was born. My mother took me to church in her womb. I was a "comfortable" Christian. I had not heard of present-day healing through the power of the Holy Spirit. If I had been told, I wouldn't have believed it!

In 1995, my wife was diagnosed with a condition called peripheral neuropathy. Essentially, the nerves in her legs, feet, arms and hands were withering. It was untreatable, according to the doctor.

In early July, 1997, I went to the altar a for healing prayer for my wife, at St. Paul's United Methodist Church of the Voyager, in Coronado, California. There, Harold and Ginny Weeks prayed for her. They suggested to me that my wife come to the healing classes at the church on Wednesdays at 7 p.m. Harold said, "What do you have to lose?" I couldn't refute the logic. I sincerely wanted my wife to be healed. That night, I suggested to my wife that she go to the class. At the same time, two others in the church also suggested that she go. She went. I stayed home. When she came home, she woke me up to tell me that she saw strange things happening. She saw arms and legs changing length!! I found it hard to believe. However, I knew that she would not tell me something that was not true.

The second week, she said that her arms had moved! It had happened while a person had prayed for her! This was too much for me. I had to see what was going on!

At the next meeting, I was shocked and amazed by what I saw. By the power of hands-on prayer, calling upon Jesus and the Holy Spirit, people had their arms and legs shortened and lengthened. They fell down, under the power of the Holy Spirit. I couldn't believe it was happening. It was staggering to me! No one I had ever known had said that this was possible, through Jesus.

All through church as a youth, the Boy Scouts at church, and as an adult in church (I was then 56 years old) I had never even heard of the healing power of the Holy Spirit!

In August, I went back the second time. I started listening intently to what was being prayed. Each person said things a different way. It was disconcerting that I could find no one mantra or prayer that healed. Was there a pattern that called down the power of the Holy Spirit? There was!

I found that the healing class members would first call on the authority of Jesus Christ. Then, they would command the injured part of the body to be healed. There were different ways to describe the injury or sickness. There were different ways to command the body to be healed. Sometimes specific systems of the body would be commanded. Sometimes the prayers were more general. However, this pattern was always the same.

Harold Weeks, the facilitator, always had books and tapes available on how to heal. My wife and I started borrowing more and more. I started listening to about one tape a day, as I was dressing, eating, or exercising. Becky listened to several each week. I started studying Bible verses, like Mark 16:16-18. It said believers would heal the sick and cast out demons. I read John 14:14. It said that, "You may ask me for anything in my name, and I will do it." This was good news! Anyone who was a believer could heal the sick and cast out demons! What a revelation this was to me? The church had not shared that secret!

After the third meeting, I started to "practice" on myself. I was amazed that my body responded to my own prayers for healing. I had a pain in my ankle. I commanded it to leave, and it did. While watching videotapes by Charles and Frances Hunter, Frances told how she got rid of headaches. I tried it and it worked! I got rid of headaches three times that week. By the third time, all I had to do was raise my hand towards my head and the pain left. I was learning about spiritual warfare!

Yes, I found that our, "pain," was caused by an evil spirit! Whoa! Satan is on earth? Causing me pain. Yes! I got rid of my headaches by casting out a demon I just said "Out, in the name of Jesus!"

This was another revelation to me. In the church, we talked of Heaven and Hell. We talked of God and Satan. Never had I heard that Satan could be alive and well here on earth, causing pain, sorrow and death! Now, I had first-hand experiences with Satan! He was real, in my life. I already had the picture that Jesus was a real force in today's world, by the healing. But when I learned that the other side, Satan, was also in today's world, I knew that the Bible, as God's word, was completely true!

I asked to be baptized by Jesus in the Holy Spirit in the next class. In the September 5, 1997, healing class, another student prayed for me to receive the power of the Holy Spirit. I received it! Hallelujah! I don't remember everything about it. Some things I remember, that my wife told me. In any case, the things told me were consistent with the things that I remembered. (But that is another story.) At the end of the evening, I started speaking in tongues, just like it says in Mark 16:17-18! Believers could do what Jesus said that they would do! My experiences had proved it to me!

By now, I was taking the Bible even more seriously. I started reading and listening to the Bible for specific thing to do and not to do. Harold said that he was trying not to "overdose" me. I told him that I didn't think that he could! He still hasn't, and I'm still listening to several tapes a week. Some tapes more than once. Now that I know that this is about either damnation or salvation, I can't afford to be wrong! I want to spend eternity with Jesus! I sure don't want to go to Hell!

On November 10, 1997, I tried some major healing. I had an enlarged prostate, which was a real problem for me. I was getting up at night four and five times. It disrupted my sleep. I lost sleep. I had been taking saw palmetto, with good results. However, I was out of pills. I got some more, $60.00 worth. When I got them home, I thought, "Why use them when I could just call on the Holy Spirit?"

Yes, you guessed it. I prayed that night just before going to sleep. The next morning, I realized that I didn't have to get up during the night to go to the bathroom! From that day on, I have not had to take any more saw palmetto. I had received a major healing by the Holy Spirit answering my prayer, just like it says in John 14:14, quoted above. I, as a believer, had asked, and Jesus sent his Holy Spirit to do the job. Thank you, Jesus!

I knew that according to the Bible, I was saved and could expect to go to Heaven when I die. That was because I had received the Power of the Holy Spirit. I knew that, because I had received the Gift of Healing. However, I felt that something was lacking. I didn't know what. Hold on, I was about to find out!

I was introduced to Ed and Millie. They have a charismatic ministry at the Hotel in San Diego every second Friday at 7 p.m. We had started to go there, my wife and I. We attended the December 12, 1997, service it had great meaning for me (but that is another story!).

By the next morning, I started to have a feeling of great joy surge in my heart. It got greater and greater. On the third day I knew in my heart that I was born again! Jesus' power authority is great! Hallelujah!

At that time, I asked my wife to marry me again. She said YES (Thank you, Jesus)! I asked our pastor, to re-marry us and re-baptize me. He said yes. After 35, we were remarried in Jesus Christ! Hallelujah!

Since that time, Becky and I have been so blessed, it is hard to believe. We had started a journal of the blessings and healing early on. It was a good thing. Now, we can read them over and over. We have earnestly prayed to turn control of our lives over to Jesus, to be obedient to Jesus, to tithe, to follow the Commandments, and to use the Gifts of the Holy Spirit freely. I have a peace now that is complete. My fears of death and the future are gone. I now have, just like the song says, "Blessed Assurance." Hallelujah!

In February 1998, I went in for an annual physical at a Kaiser HMO facility. I was told by the physician that I had a score of "14" on the PSA test. That level had risen from "2.5," about five years earlier. The doctor said that there was a good chance that I had cancer of the prostate. I had to take a second, more specific test.

Before I took the more specific test, I went to Ed & Millie Jolley's services. They held prayer for me and against cancer, on March 13, 1998. The next Monday, I went in for the second test. The test results had "no medical significance." HALLELUJAH! Thank you JESUS!

If you want more of what Jesus has for you, stick a toe in the water. Want to get rid of pain, suffering, fear, and sickness? Want to live forever in heaven?

*"When the sun was setting, all those who had any that were sick with various diseases brought them to Him; and He laid His hands on every one of them and healed them." Luke 4:40*

# The Testimony of Frank Leslie

May 25, 1995 presented me with quite a surprise, and another of life's challenges. Confronted with the evidence of a Grade IV malignant brain tumor, my experience of life soon changed. Surgery, radiation, and a shortened chemotherapy regimen left me physically and emotionally exhausted. Against my doctor's wishes, I stopped taking chemotherapy in January 1996. There is no medical "cure" for brain cancer so I set forth seeking a miracle and an opportunity to serve a God that might graciously heal me. Throughout my life I had often wondered about God—His existence, nature, and purpose for us. Unfortunately, I had never comfortably resolved these questions. This was soon to change.

In February 1996, my wife and I attended our first Christian healing class led by Hal Weeks. Just hearing about such a class affected me profoundly. Very shortly, we witnessed the power of God's Spirit in our lives. We began to immerse ourselves in the literature and practice of "hands on healing," intercessory prayer, etc. The manifestations of God's love and power brought great comfort to us. Despite a reoccurrence of the tumor (Grade II) in March 1996, my faith and thankfulness continued to grow as God used me to help others. For one year the recurrent tumor remained. In March 1997, the area in which the tumor was clear—and remains so to this day. Thankful for the steadfast prayers of many and the power of God's Holy Spirit invoked through the name of

Jesus, this testimony is in service to God so that others might seek a personal relationship with His Son Jesus and receive this blessing.

*"Beloved, I wish above all things that thou mayest prosper and be in health, even as thy soul prospereth."*
*3 John 2*

# My Appointment for A Miracle
## By
## Dr. Jim Strickhausen

At that very moment, 1:07 p.m., I was closing my briefcase, turning off my computer, and preparing to leave the church office. I attempted to rise from my chair, but the lower half of my body would not move. I tried again and again but it was as if I was glued to the chair. "A.m. I having another stroke?" Fear began to grip me. I was already partially paralyzed in my left arm. I had dull crushing chest pains that are common and parts of my upper body had become numb and weak. Was I now becoming TOTALLY paralyzed? Suddenly someone opened my office door and what felt like a strong gust of wind rushed into my face.

To fully understand what I'm sharing here, I must go back in time to a pastor's retreat near Chattanooga, TN in the early 1980's. Dr Bill Hamon, a respected New Testament prophet, spoke a prophetic word over my life as he was laying hands on me in prayer. The Holy Spirit spoke through him that God was going to anoint me for the healing ministry. The prophecy said that I would preach a little, stop, lay hands on the sick, preach a little more, then stop again and lay hands on the sick. He prophesied that not only healing would occur, but that mighty miracles would take place as well. As the years progressed, other reputable men and women of God prophesied of this healing ministry that the Lord would give me.

Over the next few years the Lord whispered over and over again to my heart that I would profoundly impact my generation. Since my personality is conservative, I kept all these prophecies and dealings from the Lord to myself, sharing them only with my precious wife, Dina, who has been my encourager, friend, and confidant for over twenty one years.

In the early 1990's I was on one of many trips to Mexico, when a Mexican pastor's wife, sister laid hands on me and prophesied that I would travel to far away places to minister to many people. I wondered how this would be possible? But within a few short years, my wife and I traveled to Russia, Romania, Italy, and back to Mexico. We witnessed people receiving Jesus, and witnessed supernatural healing-taking place.

However, in 1996, my health began to decline. I began to experience classic signs of "burn out." For years I was an "over-achiever." Actually, to be perfectly honest, I was addicted to work. As a workaholic, my day began at 4:00 a.m. and often ended late into the night. My self-esteem was tied to the number of hours I worked, and what I could accomplished in those hours. Slowly but surely I was killing myself. Having served as a senior pastor for a number of years and now serving as the associate pastor for church administration, counseling, and the missions department, I easily became immersed in my work. The doctors told me that if I didn't slow down and take a sabbatical, I would be dead within five years.

My dear friend, and the senior pastor of our church, insisted that I take a nine-month sabbatical beginning April 1, 1997. After strongly resisting, I realized that Pastor Bob was not going to relent, so I submitted to his request. The nine months went by very fast and it was indeed a time of mental and emotional healing. I was faced with the reality that I had put my work first and my family second. But rather than focusing on the past, I chose to repent and make the most of the present.

January 1998 arrived too soon, and I was back at work. I worked hard at limiting my hours so as not to repeat my past habits and propensity for being a workaholic. During a Sunday morning service in January, our worship pastor and a recognized prophet, suddenly stopped in the middle of the worship service and began to prophesy that God was adding years to my life and that the next millennium was mine. The prophecy further stated that I would be traveling to many places and hundreds, even thousands, would be healed in a single service. There was a heavy weight of God's presence and quickening in that moment, and I was reminded of the prophecies of years past which I had kept secret.

But as the year progressed, it seemed the exact opposite was happening to me. My blood pressure, or Refractory Essential Hypertension, soared to dangerous levels. The doctors were very alarmed because none of the medications to lower blood pressure had any effect. My health was deteriorating rapidly, and I became concerned, but was in a state of denial too. I started experiencing numbness and weakness in my left arm and I had dull crushing pains in my chest. A degree of paralysis was setting in on the upper left side of my body. My doctor rushed me to several specialists for blood work, EKGs, two MRIs, X-rays, and a renal angiogram. As expected, the tests confirmed a mild heart attack and a mini-stroke. That day I went home and wept bitterly.

As bad went to worse, and all my doctors from Huntsville to Mobile insisted that I retire immediately. They said my heart and body needed sustained physical rest and the minimum amount of stress. Dina and I discussed it and agreed that I would officially retire the end of May 1999. My heart was heavy. I felt that all my hopes and dreams for ministering to people were gone. We resigned ourselves to looking for a small house in a small town where I would spend the balance of my life. Hopelessness and feelings of futility wrapped themselves around me. But God had plans for us, and on April 7, I had a miraculous personal encounter with the Holy Spirit. Putting this encounter into print doesn't begin to do justice to what actually happened, but I believe it will encourage you in your faith nonetheless. So here we go!

Dr. Bob Hellmann, the senior pastor of our church, was upstairs in his prayer room. I did not know that he was praying for me, and my, condition of ill health. At precisely 1:07 p.m., as he was speaking to the Lord, the Holy Spirit interrupted him. The Spirit spoke concisely, "JIM IS HEALED!" This was not just Bob believing promises from the Bible that I was healed; rather this was the voice of God speaking with finality and urgency that I was ALREADY healed. The Spirit DID NOT say that I was GOING TO BE healed, but that I WAS healed! As Pastor Bob basked in the glory of the Spirit's majestic voice, the Spirit spoke again, commanding him to go down stairs and tell me what had just happened. He quickly glanced at his watch and said, "Holy Spirit, don't let Jim leave before I get to him."

As I sat there frozen to my chair and unable to move, Bob entered my office at around 1:10 p.m. When he entered, a mysterious yet wonderful wind rushed into my face. Instantly, I knew the Holy Spirit had come in a special way. Pastor Bob stood in front of my desk and rehearsed to me what the Spirit said to him at 1:07 p.m., "JIM IS HEALED!" I remember well that Bob's face was radiating with the brightness of God's presence.

Then he began to pray and thank God for what He had just done. He requested that I get up from my chair and come to the other side of the desk. Without even thinking of my then present, "CAN'T MOVE CRISIS", I bolted out of the chair, walked to the other side, and sat in another chair.

You would have to know Pastor Bob and his entire family to understand what I'm about to say. His hands are, without fail, very cold to the touch. Those cold hands now were touching me as he began praying again, simply thanking God for what He had already done. My eyes were closed as I felt those cold hands on my left shoulder and arm, where I was partially paralyzed and numb. But then, suddenly, he placed his hands over my heart in the middle of my chest. Now his hands were hot, even blazing. I just knew my skin must have been burning. After removing his hands, my chest continued to burn intensely. As I repeatedly touched my chest, I felt the heat leap into my hands and I reveled in the intensity of the anointing. (Even as I write this testimony, my chest is hot again in the exact place Bob's hands had been upon me.)

There in the office, Bob instructed me to move my left arm. The first time, the movement was very limited, but each time I moved it, my arm became stronger and the pain grew milder. Never had I experienced the presence of the Holy Spirit so strongly. I could actually feel the Spirit of God penetrating my inmost being and every cell in my body. While this was happening, Bob received a vision from the Lord. He saw me being attended to by the Lord himself, like medics attending to someone at the scene of an accident. Then prophetic words began pouring out of his mouth. The prophecy stated that the curse of death had been reversed and God was adding 33 years to my life. The message continued that the healing anointing that had once been felt in my hands and flowed out to the people for instantaneous miracles was returning to me, and that my primary focus would be that of a "Healing Minister" and less of an administrator. I would be going to the nations of the world to lay hands on the sick, and many miracles would take place. Countries that were mentioned during this heavily anointed prophecy were Mexico, Costa Rica, Russia, Romania, and India. Other nations would also be included. Money would be no problem, the Spirit continued, telling me that I should never think that there wouldn't be enough. Rather, the money would flow in freely and there would be more than enough.

After the prophetic word ended, I was able to share with Pastor Bob, for the first time, the many similar prophecies that I had received over the previous twenty years. They all lined up with this fresh prophetic word. The difference was that previous prophecies spoke of the future, whereas this prophecy spoke of NOW.

Later, after this incredible encounter, I realized that many things had taken place that day in my office and that I was unaware of at the time. The Holy Spirit had delivered me from the driving force of a big demon named "workaholic." All my life this demon had driven me to work from 4:00 a.m. every morning to late at night, every day. This constant "driven feeling" was indeed driving me somewhere—to my grave! It deceived me into thinking that I must work all the time to be a success and to have high self-esteem. Praise God, that demon is gone! I am a different person altogether. For the first time in my life, I can relax and rest without self-condemnation.

Two days after my miracle appointment, while at home, I was rubbing my left shoulder and arm. Immediately, I noticed that all the numbness was completely gone. I even pinched myself in several places; all the feeling had returned.

My next appointment was with a neurologist. He wanted to run a certain test to classify the stroke and find exactly where it had occurred. The test took about 45 minutes. The neurologist became very puzzled. He said he could find absolutely no sign of a stroke.

So he wanted to perform a MRI to see if I had a pinch nerve. But I told him I had recently had two MRIs before my healing and they did not reveal any pinch nerves. I told him the reason he couldn't find anything was because God had supernaturally healed me.

Of course all of my doctors including the neurologist had been advising me not to do anything strenuous. However, after leaving that neurologist's office, I was so excited about the report, that when I returned to the parking garage, I couldn't remember where I parked my car. Without thinking, I ran up five flights of stairs in search of it. Then, when I got home, I decided to mow the grass. Upon finishing, I had no shortness of breath, no chest pain, and zero fatigue. I was totally and completely healed indeed!

Many months have gone by since God healed me. Concerning my blood pressure, doctors had once said, "It's impossible for you to be living." Now all my blood tests are perfectly normal. For many years, I had the type of high blood pressure that wouldn't even respond to dangerously high dosages of medicine. But after my miracle appointment with the Holy Spirit, the doctor kept reducing the dosage. Finally,

I was getting dizzy on the lowest dosage and the doctor told me I no longer needed any medication. My strength and youthful vigor has returned. My daily schedule is again busy but not rushed. I am no longer internally driven by a workaholic demon. It is so good to be relaxed and enjoying life to its fullest.

In conclusion, let me say, I feel my life has just begun, and doors of ministry are opening everyday. Where would I be without the precious Holy Spirit sent from the Father by Jesus? Where would I be without a caring, praying pastor? Where would I be without a wife who stood by my side even at the lowest point of my life? Praise Jesus! And thank you, Holy Spirit, for an appointment I will never forget!

# A Beautiful Inspirational Story
## By
## Chad

This past week was perhaps one of the most stressful weeks that I have had in my life. Stress and anxiety seemed to be coming at me from all directions and in many different shapes and forms. It started with some problems with my physical health. I have been in and out of doctors' offices for several months now trying to find out what has been causing me the pains and problems I have had with my intestines and chest. Well, it seemed they had straightened that out, but now I was having severe numbness and tightness in the entire left portion of my upper body. This is where the worrying began.

And then there were a couple of days when I had to be on the road traveling to clients, and I always get stressed when I have to drive long distances. Put on top of all of this a recent decision my wife and I made to start looking for a house, and you have one stressed-out person.

I regret that I did not find this verse in the Bible earlier in the week. But in some way, I think perhaps I had. The only thing that was able to get me through the week was daily giving my worry and stress over to my gentle father Jesus Christ. Each morning, I prayed much the same words as the Psalmist recorded here at the beginning of Psalm 57. Of course, my words were not quite as eloquent, but they had the same meaning. I simply asked that God watch over me in the coming hours of the day ahead and that I was laying all of my burdens upon him, trusting that he would take care of them.

My pastor once said that you could tell the size of your God by looking at the size of your worry list. The longer your list is the smaller your God. God tells us time and time again in his word that we should not worry, and that he will take care of us. In Matthew 6:25 he tells us, "do not worry," and again in Philippians 4:6 we are told to "be anxious for nothing." But our human nature causes us to hold on to all of these worries and anxieties that can bring us nothing but harm.

I have come to realize that no matter how well our life may be going, we will always have problems and concerns. There are always going to be things to "worry" about. But if we will do as the psalmist says and take refuge in the shadow of our God, we can rest there until all of the worries and calamities have passed us by. I recently received an e-mail about a "worry tree." The essence of the story was that each day as the man came home from work he would pause before going into his house, and "hang" his worries on the little tree beside of the front door. He discovered that when he would come out the next morning, there were not nearly as many worries as he had left the night before. Well as God's creatures we have the greatest worry tree of all. We can give our worries over to him each morning or evening, and he will bear them for us.

So in the coming week, let's give our worries to God and see how much better our week goes. He will take them all, no matter what. Whether it is a concern over a big sales presentation, finishing a big project, choosing the right house to buy, or even just choosing what to fix for dinner each night, God will take care of it.

Chad Janey
Charlotte, NC, USA

# Miracles Still Happen

Today I have the privilege of praying for Irena's father, Michael. Upon our arrival Michael complained about the incredible pain in his fingers. Things had gotten so bad that he could hardly hold a knife or fork. The joints were so badly deformed. I asked Michael to place his hand on the table. As I placed my hands over his I prayed for healing-nothing happened. Suddenly I felt a tingling from the top of my head to the tips of my fingers and I commanded the spirit of arthritis to leave his hands. After I had finished praying I told Michael to cry out to Jesus to help him, and this he did. Then I asked him to raise his hands and praise God for his healing. After Michael had finished praising God, he told me that he had also felt God's anointing from the top of his head to the tips of his fingers. Before prayer, the fingers had been icy cold and stiff, but now they were visibly perspiring and Michael could move then without pain. Praise God for a mighty miracle.

### Healed of Hemophilia

As the grandfather and mother of my student sat opposite me during the parent interview, I informed them that the child's progress was not satisfactory. Their response shocked me. "Don't you know he suffers from hemophilia? That is why he is absent from school so much." I could have slid under the table with embarrassment. On one of the rare occasions when he was in class, I decided to pray for him. As I stood near him, I prayed this simple prayer in my mind. Oh Lord, my God, please drain all the imperfect blood out of him, and fill him with new blood containing blood clotting cells. Lord Jesus let your blood flow through that boy's body. Then I claimed the boys total healing and wholeness, according Isaiah 53:5.

I finally realized that the child hadn't missed class for some time. I asked him how he felt. The boy told me that neither he, nor his family could understand whey he hadn't needed a blood transfusion for four weeks. Usually, at least one transfusion a week would have been necessary. Also, due to constant injections in the left arm, the muscles had wasted away. He was totally amazed that I had prayed for his healing and that God in fact had worked a miracle. Praise God, when Jesus healed the blood condition, he also restored the muscles in the left arm.

### Gods Healing Power

Next, I was taken to another village to pray for two women who had been sent home from hospital to die. One had throat cancer and the other breast cancer. Jerry and Pastor Lucas, plus other people from their village had accompanied us. Both women were housed in the same hut. After I had greeted the women and their relatives, I requested that, everybody who was not a firm believer should leave the hut. In the end, only Jerry, Pastor Lucas, the two patients and I were left. I asked the Holy Spirit to tell me how to pray and to anoint my hands with Jesus' healing power. The mighty presence of God was felt in that hut as I prayed. In each case, I was given a different prayer, based upon the Bible.

God performed a mighty miracle of healing in both women, but now certain principles needed to be followed in the natural. The Bible tells us that, "To have faith is to be sure of things we hope for, to be certain of the things we cannot see." So in my heart I believed that the women were healed, but their wasted bodies indicated otherwise. So God instructed me to say the following to the relatives and friends of the patients, who had once again entered the hut—Time was needed for the wasted bodies to repair. First of all, the smoking fire was to be put out and the cooking was to be done outside the hut. Every morning, or afternoon, the women were to be carried out into the sun and fresh air. Although I only have a limited knowledge of nutrition, God gave me some amazing ideas on healthy light meals. The food items were all easily available in, or around the village. After all, when Jesus raised the little girl from the dead, the first thing he did was to tell the parents to feed her.

Pastor Lucas interpreted in Pidgin what I had said. The husband from the woman who had suffered from throat cancer then started a lively discussion. Although I could only speak a few words of Pidgin, God interpreted the conversation for me and I found myself saying, "Stop." How dare you, say that your wife cannot eat because her throat has been eaten up by the cancer?

God is a mighty God, who can and already has repaired the damage done to your wife's throat. Everybody stared at me in horror because they knew that I did not understand the language and only God could have told me what was going on. My words did much to destroy the man's unbelief. After my stay in the Highlands, I was invited to go for four days to Madang. Agnus had invited me to visit her mother and stepfather in the settlement. Here again God combined the supernatural with the physical in a mighty way.

Marlies Zechner, Sydney, Australia (http//www.christian-faith.com)

> *"Truly, truly, I say to you, he who believes in Me, the works that I do shall he do also; and greater {works} than these shall he do; because I go to the Father. And whatever you ask in My name, that will I do, that the Father may be glorified in the Son." (NAS)*
> John 14:12-13

# I HAVE IT, CANCER
By
## Pastor Harold Weeks

In July 1971, at the age of 58, I discovered a lump in my left groin about the size of a large olive. This was diagnosed to be a lymphoma or cancer of the lymphatic system. It was treated with cobalt for a period of 21 one days. I continued to have periodic check-ups until early in 1975. As time went on I discovered several nodes in my neck and under my right arm that seemed to be growing. In August 1977, at the age of 64, a large node was removed from my right armpit. It was diagnosed as a poorly differentiated nodular lymphoma. I was then referred to an oncologist for treatment. However, he agreed to defer any treatment on the basis of my belief that I had been healed. I was scheduled to return in three months. When I returned, he could find no evidence of the cancer. He said, "If I were examining you for the first time, I would have diagnosed you as not having the disease." I continued having periodic check-ups until August 1982, at age 69, at which time he transferred me back to my family doctor. I am now 87 years old.

I believe what I initially received was the manifestation of the Baptism in the Holy Spirit. Having always believed in prayer, I had been asking God to heal me all during the course of this disease.

However, since I had not revealed my condition to more than a couple of friends, I had not received much…if any…in general prayer. For several years, I did believe I had been healed and I did receive what the, I now believe this was the deciding factor in my seeking the experience known in charismatic and Pentecostal circles as the baptism in the Holy Spirit. I received prayer for this and doctors called it a marvelous remission. But with the recurrence and the diagnosis that the condition was now serious, I became deeply troubled. At a Full Gospel Businessmen's Fellowship meeting on August 18, 1977, at the age of 64, which I had been attending for several weeks. Nothing seemed to happen at the time, but I was assured I had received this baptism and I thanked God for His gift. At about 10:30 p.m. the following Saturday evening, while in bed reading some charismatic testimonies and reflecting on them, my attention was drawn to a strange tingling sensation in my right arm. This subsided but shortly I noticed the same sensation on the side of my face. As I began to rub my face, I felt a sort of electrifying of my right arm. I remember exclaiming, "Lord, your hand is holding my hand." At that point, waves of an almost indescribable power began to sweep through my entire body. I have had similar sensations since but never again with that intensity. Yet, for several days afterwards, the power of God was so strong on me that I finally had to ask God to "lead me beside the still waters." I did then experience some abatement for a time of rest, but this was the beginning of a whole new way of life and the beginning of a new relationship with Jesus that I had never known before. At the time it was impressed on my mind that I had received three prizes. The third prize was the healing of cancer; the second prize was the deliverance from fear and doubt; and the first prize was going from knowing about Jesus to knowing Jesus as Lord. Although medical science classifies this a spontaneous remission, I claim it as a divine healing. (www.home.san.rr.com/healing/)

*"And Jesus went about all the cities and villages, teaching in their synagogues, and preaching the gospel of the kingdom, and healing every sickness and every disease among the people"*
*Matthew: 9:35*

# Valerie Smith's Healing Testimony

In 1996, I was walking home late at night and stumbled over the side-walk, falling off a pair of high heel boots. I tore the ligament connecting to my right ankle. Thinking it was just a sprain, I did not seek immediate medical attention. After one year the ankle was still not properly healed and caused me quite a lot of pain at the end of each day. I sought help from a sports-injury specialist. His prognosis was grim: the original tissue was damaged beyond repair. He offered me a grue-some option of surgery that would cut a good tendon, drill holes through the bone and weave the tendon through to re-secure the ankle. I chose not to take the option.

Also, my lower back, hips, and both knees had been badly affected by two car accidents in 1996, and quite often they cause me pain and difficulty in movement.

Then in 1998, God told me in prayer that He would restore all that the enemy has stolen and that I was to expect total restoration of my mind and body.

This past year looked like things were getting worse in my lower limbs instead of better. The swelling and stiffness in my right ankle and both knees were a daily problem; I went to the altar for prayer almost every Sunday and the pain and stiffness would dissipate, but the relief lasted only a few days.

A few months ago, my pastor began teaching us that faith is an action, not just a passive state of agreement with the word. He said that the confessions of your mouth should be in harmony with your faith…not on the obvious circumstances before you.

I began to declare out loud the promise God gave me in prayer and also to speak out loud some verses in the Bible that pertained to my problem. Getting ready in the morning became an easier task as the pain and stiffness left, but it was still a daily battle to get relief.

On August 3, 1999—A married couple from St. Paul's United Methodist Church in Coronado, California is visiting my church. They notice my limp, and asked me if I would like prayer for my ankle. To my knowledge the couple were not pastors, elders, or visiting evangelists with world renown healing ministries. I said "O.K., sure," without seriously expecting anything more than some relief from the swelling and pain. What I didn't know about them was that this couple places great faith in Jesus' words in Mark 16:18b: "and they will lay hands on the sick, and they will recover."

When the couple began to pray and lay their hands on my ankle, the power of the Holy Spirit came over me so strongly that I could no longer sit upright in my chair. As I was gently slumping over to the ground, a strong thought entered my mind. It was so strong that I spoke it out loud: "Expect something great." Then the verse Matthew 7:11 came to me and I asked Bill to read it out loud to me from his bible. "If you being evil know how to give good gifts to your children, how much more will your Father in heaven give good gifts to those who ask Him?" The words pierced through me and I wept uncontrollably. Another resounding thought filled me "Yes, this is the day". I grabbed hold of that thought and responded "yes" several times in reply and I knew that this was really it. I spent the next three hours lying on the floor as the couple prayed and lightly kept their hands on me. In about a half an hour, the wife said that the swelling was completely gone and a new phase of healing began.

Another loud thought inside my head said that a new ligament was being formed. When I spoke the thought out loud to the couple, something amazing happened. My right leg shot straight up into the air; the muscles began to flutter by themselves much like a guitar string vibrates. At the same time that happened, a wave of laughter flew out of my mouth from deep within my belly as if I had heard a funny joke. As long as the muscles fluttered, I continued to laugh. Then a soft peace filled me and everything relaxed for a while. A young lady waiting to lock up the church walked over and asked me how it was going. I answered softly "I have a new ligament," and then the fluttering began all over again.

When the peace came back; Bill asked if my left knee was giving me trouble and I replied, "yes." This began a different phase of healing much like chiropractic adjustment but without a human chiropractor. My hips turned this way and that way by themselves without anyone touching them. I heard and felt several vertebrae in my lower back, mid-back, and my neck go back into place. I felt no more pain or stiffness in any area!

I am writing this approximately one month after the event. My ankle is completely whole, and I am in the process of rebuilding muscle tissue daily. I am still amazed at the faithfulness of God. "He who started a good work in you shall be faithful to complete it." (Phil. 1:6) My lower back still sometimes goes out of place causing problems with my knees, but what is that to a God who can regenerate a severed and dead ligament? I wait with anticipation for Him to complete the work of restoration. Thank you for the opportunity to testify of the greatness of God.

Valerie Smith

*"And the people, when they knew it, followed him: and he received them, and spake unto them of the kingdom of God, and healed them that had need of healing."*
*Luke: 9:11*

# Frances Howard's Testimony

On June 4, 1993, as I was walking off of a marine dock, my life changed dramatically. A large surge hit the floating dock. The ramp, which rested on the dock, and led up to the shore was tossed up. In a flash, the several ton ramp crashed down on my foot and trapped me.

The pain was excruciating. I felt as if I was being sucked into a black hole and drained of life. I began screaming, "God, please help me! Please help me Lord!" Many on-lookers raced to help lift the ramp and pull me out. But the weight was too much. I heard fragments of sentences...discussion of how to free me...amputation." I was later told I cried out for everyone to pray. As quickly as it happened, a large surge hit the dock a second time and I was pulled free.

A doctor and a nurse ran down the ramp and took over until the rescue squad arrived. The nurse said she and the doctor were foot specialists and would administer my needs. I believe they were there to "minister" to my needs. They could not be located following my injury. They could not be located by the doctors in the hospital or by an article in the local paper. Could God have sent the second surge to free me as well as the angels to assist me? There is no doubt in my mind. The crush injury kept me in the hospital over a week. There was fear of losing the foot, and then the fear of skin grafts, and the fear of not walking again. None of these fears prevailed. I did however develop a nerve disorder referred to as Reflex Sympathetic Dystrophy.

It is an extremely painful condition that is something like putting an ice cube on an exposed nerve or having hot sauce run through your veins. There are no cures—just trial and error treatments.

After several months, my husband and I moved to San Diego. I continued with physical therapy and began treatment at the pain clinic. My husband and I started attending St. Paul's United Methodist Church in Coronado—yet another blessing. Like a vine, God was weaving a path and leading me to Him. For months we sat in the balcony where I could cry and release my emotions undetected. The pain in my foot was taking over. I was exhausted physically and emotionally. I contemplated suicide. Yet, I still felt drawn to church and found some peace when surrounded by the beautiful music.

Something we had not observed in the Methodist church before was healing prayer at the rail following communion. Some great impulse (!) sent me there, and with my husband by my side. I wanted the minister to pray for me. But as God would have it, Hal and his wife asked me to come forward. As I knelt at the rail they asked about my condition and need for prayer. I asked for "endurance of the pain." Hal responded, "we're not going to pray for endurance, but to be rid of the pain!" And in the name of Jesus as Hal touched my head, boom!

I was laying on the floor in the most wonderful tranquility and lightness. My foot was tingling. Tears started to flow and I knew something was happening, but something I didn't understand but could trust completely.

As I lay on the floor, I could see my husband's questioning face as he leaned against the front pew. I knew what he was thinking. What's going on here? And if I had suspected what was going to happen, I doubt I would have gone for healing prayer. I didn't believe those preachers I had occasionally seen on TV. Well believe me! Jesus has given authority for others to practice what He demonstrated. And what a wonderful blessing!

My pain was reduced significantly. It was not a total healing. However, I still believe that He will heal my foot one hundred percent.

However, what He gave me has changed my life. He has gotten my attention. And now I have an ongoing relationship with Him. The peace of knowing God as my Father and Jesus as my Savior weaves through every part of my life. His vine continues to grow with me, as long as I seek Him.

I am so thankful that I can walk, that God is using Hal and others from the healing class to convey His word and promises to His children, that I am being led to meaningful and fulfilling tasks. Currently I am a volunteer at a neonatal intensive care unit. I feed, rock, and diaper, and sing to premature babies. I pray for them and their families. I love my work. I pray that it is satisfying to my Father for He has given me so much. Something I would not have sought became my miracle and blessing. I know that God wants to share such with you. Seek Him for healing—whether physical or emotional.

As you stay in His word and develop an intimate relationship with Him, you will find your blessings too.

Frances Howard

# Mary Lou Luckett's Healing

In August 1998, my mammogram indicated there was a spot that looked suspicious. The doctor sent me to have a core biopsy. The report came back positive. Thereupon the surgeon recommended an excisional biopsy to remove the cancer tissue and cells. A recent pathologist's report stated that there was no residual tumor so radiation may not be necessary.

Through this whole procedure, I was upheld in prayer by, our minister, friends, and family with their prayers, love, support, and concern. I knew God was in charge and felt His presence during this entire procedure. I am optimistic that God will continue His healing process and that I am going to be all right.

"Fear not for I am with you; be not dismayed, for I am your God. I will strengthen you, yes, I will help you, I will uphold you with My righteous right hand." (Isaiah 41:10)

*"To another faith by the same spirit; to another the gifts of healing by the same Spirit'*
*1Cor: 12:9*

# Fran Bassett's
# Testimony of a Divine Healing

In the early 1970's, a friend and I had planned a trip to Hawaii. Shortly before we were to leave, I suffered a heart attack. The trip was delayed for many weeks.

When I was finally able to get my doctor's permission to leave, my friend and I set out on an amazing journey.

While vacationing there, we came across an announcement about a visiting evangelist named Vaneta, and decided we would like to attend her meeting.

The next night, we drove down to Kahalui to find her. After a fruitless search, we gave up and returned to our borrowed home on the mountainside.

Not wanting to miss her, we drove down the next night. We were met by a darkened building and by a dark parking lot. No light was visible anywhere. Just as we were about to leave, another car arrived. They, too, were looking for her. Being natives of Kahalui, they knew of another building on the campus and soon guided us to it. Sure enough, there was light from a single bulb in a hallway! Making our way to it, we were soon surrounded by others who had come to hear Vaneta.

At the end of the session, my friend and I joined the healing line. As I approached Vaneta she exclaimed, "Where have you been? I have been looking for you." The next thing I remember was my friend was on her knees beside me (I had fallen under the power of the Holy Spirit) saying to the evangelist, "She has a heart problem." Veneta's reply was, "Not anymore."

And sure enough, God had reached down and healed my life-long disease of rheumatic fever. Gone were the painful, swollen, joints. The enlarged heart began shrinking and my doctor subsequently cancelled my medication.

I was and still am healed through the caring of an intercessor, and by the power of the Holy Spirit, in the name of Jesus. Alleluia!

Fran Bassett

*"Behold, I will bring it health and cure, and I will cure them, and will reveal unto them the abundance of peace and truth."*
*Jeremiah: 33:6*

# TESTIMONY OF MS. W.C.L.

August 1998

A few weeks ago, my heart went bad. I had a diagnosis of arterial fibrillation. I was in the hospital emergency twice in less than two weeks. The first time I blacked out, and was taken to the hospital emergency. I was given all the treatment a heart patient gets, the machines, wires, and patches, etc. The cardiologist was called in. He put me on a blood thinner and other medications. He told me there was a 2-out-of-3 chance I would have a stroke before morning! The cardiologist came in the next morning. He looked at the blood test, and checked me over. My heart was back to normal. The blood thinner was working, I could go home and continue all medication. I was warned: If there was any pain around my heart, any weakness, to get to emergency quick! He would see me in 2 weeks otherwise. I was home three to four days and started to bleed inside. I went back to emergency. The doctor didn't know where the blood was coming from, but they did know they couldn't stop it. The blood had to be thickened and that would take time. So they did blood test all night, like every two hours until the blood thickened. I was released from the hospital with warning: don't pick up a knife, don't shave your legs, don't ride in a car etc. If I cut myself or fell and hurt myself, they could not stop the blood.

I was told to stay in the house until the blood stopped. I was released from the hospital on Friday. I noticed on Saturday, that the blood was less.

Then Sunday morning there was hardly any blood. So I said, "I'm going to church." I had to walk about 2-3 blocks, but I felt I could make it. I wore flat shoes and walked slow and I made it. I always sit in the same seat in church each Sunday, with a friend. She already knew about my heart problem and was asking me about my health, when a friend of hers stopped to say hello to her.

This is when I met Becky Hitt. My friend asked me to tell Becky about my heart problem. I did. It was close to time for church services to start. Becky was going to sit in another spot. But she said to me, "I will pray for you!" (At this time I didn't know that Becky did healing prayer). I thanked her. I thought she meant she would remember me in her prayers next week. I thought what a kind nice lady she was to pray for me. I sure needed all the prayer I could get!

So I sat through the services, but began to get very tired, and little pains were all around my heart. The doctor has told me this might happen. If so, I was to get to emergency fast. I thought I was on my way. I was leaving my seat when Becky, the Prayer Lady, came and touched me on the arm. She said, "my husband Bill and I would like to pray for you." She caught me off-guard. I liked the idea of prayer very much. But I didn't know it was to be now, in the church. And too, I had this pain all around my heart like fine needles sticking in the flesh. I was asking myself, "Should I go for home and the hospital, or prayer?" I went for the prayer! Bill and Becky prayed for me. Then Bill asked me, "How do you feel?" My mouth flew open. I said, "The pain around my heart is gone! Bill, Becky and I all said, "Praise the Lord!" I walked home a little faster than I had coming. I felt fine all the next week.

On Sunday, I waved to Bill & Becky that I was okay. Then the Friday of the next week I saw the cardiologist, for a follow-up visit. This would tell the story—what they would add to, take away, what medications I would take, etc. (I did dread this visit). The nurse saw me first and she took my blood pressure. She said, "looks good." Then the doctor did what he does, checked the pulse, lungs, then moved to the front of the chest, and then moved to the back. He would listen in one spot then move to another spot, move back and listen to the same spot again. (I would think he had found something.) When he came around where I could see his face. There was a big smile on his face, he said "Everything is just perfect. Your heart is so in tune, I could set my watch by it." Then, he said, "I'll tell you what I'm going to do? I'm going to take you off all medication, and put you on one small aspirin a day. We will try you on this, but if there's any problem, I will put you back on the other medications, but in smaller doses." I said, "Oh, no, no, the aspirin is going to be okay. Everything will be okay! For I am getting some very effective prayer for me at the church." The doctor looked at me and smiled. He said, "I will see you in six months."

Praise the Lord!

# Becky Hitt's Testimony

I used to go to church when I felt like it, or if I had enough time. I only prayed when I had a terrible problem. Sometimes, my prayer was answered, but usually it was not. I was a "911" Christian. Then in August 1994, I was diagnosed with a degenerative neurological disorder that interfered with my balance, coordination, and fine-motor control.

Some friends, including my husband, Bill, encouraged me to attend a prayer and healing class at St. Paul's United Methodist Church in July 1997. What did I have to lose? I figured it would be all right for somebody to pray for me. Nothing could have prepared me for what was to come!

I watched and listened intently for the first two meetings, marveling over the wonderful testimonies that were given. The instructor and students kept referring to the Baptism in the Holy Spirit, which I asked someone to explain. I remained confused to a degree on this, partly due to my own lack of knowledge of the Scriptures. One of the concepts I did understand was that the Holy Spirit could be invited into that room to heal someone in the name of Jesus.

During the third class, I asked for healing. The person who prayed for me asked the Holy Spirit to enter my body and provide an outward demonstration of an inner healing. He did! My arms started moving around and my body started twisting. This continued for about ten minutes. I was not causing this movement. I cried all the way home, because I had never really believed that there was a God. Now, I knew there was!

Not long after that, I learned that I was a child of God. Although I had heard this many times before, it never meant anything to me. This impacted me tremendously to know that God loved me. I had been exposed to years of verbal abuse and I never had an earthly father who loved me. I didn't even like myself. It was such a comfort to learn that God did. Unfortunately, I had a great deal of bitterness and resentment built up over the years.

I learned that God is Sovereign. He is the one who decides who, what and when someone gets cured. He knew I needed inner healing and healing of memories more than I needed the neurological problem resolved.

In the meantime, Bill and I had read everything we could on healing, baptism in the Holy Spirit and Jesus' teachings. We read God's word and continued going to the healing class. Eventually, Bill and I were both baptized in the Holy Spirit and turned our lives over to Jesus.

As the months went by, I found I could confess my sins and forgive those who had hurt me. This was necessary before physical or inner healing could occur. I went through some inner healing exercises, such as visualizing Jesus was in the room with me during some traumatic incidents in my life. The Lord dissolved my bitterness and resentfulness and I grew happier and at peace with myself. I never had liked myself, but as time went by, I not only began to like myself, I grew to feel worthy of God's love.

Jesus is the same, yesterday, today, and forever. I have discovered it is possible to enjoy heaven on earth today, with all of God's promised abundance and blessings. I have joy in my heart and the indwelling of the Holy Spirit. With God, all things are possible.

# About the Author

Linda J. Phillips is a Registered Nurse with 23 years experience in Nursing. She has experienced Heart Disease as a professional caregiver and as a patient. Linda is an accomplished painter and author. Her book "Simply Beautiful" was published in 1987. Linda was divinely inspired to write this book for the emotional support of heart patients.

# Glossary of Terms

## A

Aneurysm—An abnormal swelling of the wall of an artery, caused by a weakening in the vessel wall.

Angina pectoris—Pain experienced in the chest, arms, or jaw because of a lack of oxygen to the heart muscle.

Angioma—A tumor made of blood vessels or lymph vessels that is not cancerous.

Angioplasty—The use of surgery to make a damaged blood vessel function properly again; may involve widening or reconstructing the blood vessel.

Anticoagulants—Drugs used to stop abnormal blood clotting.

Antiemetics—Drugs used to treat nausea and vomiting.

Antihistamine—A drug that relieves an allergic reaction by stopping the effects of histamine, the substance responsible for the negative symptoms associated with the reaction.

Antihypertensives—Drugs used to relieve the symptoms and prevent the damage that can occur from high blood pressure.

Aorta—The main artery in the body carrying oxygenated blood from the heart to other arteries in the body.

Aortic stenosis—Narrowing of the opening of the aortic valve in the heart, which increases resistance to blood flow from the left ventricle to the aorta.

Arteriosclerosis—A disorder causing thickening and hardening of artery walls.

Arteritis—Inflammation of the walls of an artery, and that causes the passageway to become narrower.

Artery—A large blood vessel that carries blood from the heart, to tissues and organs in the body.

Atherectomy—A procedure performed to remove plaque that is blocking an artery.

Atheroma—Fatty deposits on the inner walls of blood vessels, which can cause narrowing and decrease blood flow.

Atherosclerosis—Narrowing of the lining of the arteries due to the accumulation of fat and other materials; leads to coronary heart disease, stroke, and other disorders

Atria—The two upper chambers of the heart; the singular form is atrium.

Atrial fibrillation—An irregular heartbeat in which the upper chambers of the heart beat inconsistently and rapidly.

Atrial flutter—An irregular heartbeat in which the upper chambers of the heart beat rapidly but consistently.

Atrial septal defect—A hole located in the wall between the two upper chambers of the heart.

# B

Balloon angioplasty—A technique that uses a balloon catheter to open arteries clogged with fatty deposits.

Balloon catheter—A hollow tube with a small, inflatable balloon at the tip, and it used to open a narrowed artery or organ that has become blocked.

Beta blocker—A type of drug used to treat high blood pressure and heart disorders by reducing the strength and rate of the pumping by the heart.

Blood clot—A semisolid mass of blood that forms to help seal and prevent bleeding; a damaged vessel.

Blood pressure—The tension in the main arteries that is created by the beating of the heart and the resistance to flow and elasticity of the blood vessels.

Blood transfusion—The transfer of blood, or any of its parts to a person who has lost blood due to an injury, disease, or operation.

Bradycardia—A slow heart rate, usually below 60 beats per minute in adults.

Bypass—A surgical technique in which the flow of blood or another body fluid is directed around a blockage.

# C

Calcification—The depositing of calcium salts in the body, which occurs normally in teeth and bones but abnormally in injured muscles and narrowed arteries.

Calcium—A plentiful mineral in the body and the basic component of teeth an bones; essential for cell function, muscle contraction, transmission of nerve impulses, and blood clotting.

Calcium channel blocker—A drug used to treat chest pain, high blood pressure, and irregular heartbeat by preventing the movement of calcium into the muscle.

Capillary—A tiny blood vessel that connects the smallest arteries to the smallest veins and allows exchange of oxygen and other materials between blood cells and body tissue cells.

Cardiac arrest—The sudden cessation of the heart's pumping action.

Cardiogenic shock—A severely dangerous condition involving decreased blood output from the heart, usually as a result of a heart attack.

Cardiomegaly—A condition marked by enlargement of the heart, either because of a thickened heart muscle or an enlarged heart chamber; usually a result of the hearthaving to work harder than normal, as occurs with high blood pressure.

Cardiomyopathy—A disease of the heart muscle that results in decreased outputand reduced blood flow.

Cardiopulmonary resuscitation—The administration of heart compression and artificial respiration to restore circulation and breathing.

Cardiopulmonary bypass—This refers to the placement of the patient onto extracorporeal membrane oxygenation. This device takes blood from the body, oxygenates via a machine and then returns it to the systemic circulation under pressure. This allows the surgeon adequate time to perform primary heart surgery on a temporarily nonfunctioning heart.

Cardiac tamponade—Interference with the venous return of blood, to the heart, and due to an extensive accumulation of blood in the pericardium (pericardial effusion).

Cardiovascular system—The heart and blood vessels that are responsible for circulating blood throughout the body.

Carditis—Inflamation of the heart.

Carotid arteries—Consists of four main arteries, that carry blood to the head and neck.

Catheter—A hollow, flexible tube inserted into the body to put in or take out fluid, or to open up or close blood vessels

Catheterization—A technique in which a hollow, flexible tube is used to drain body fluids (such as urine), to introduce fluids into the body, or to examine or widen a narrowed vein or artery.

Cholesterol—A substance in body cells that plays a role in the production of hormones and bile salts and in the transport of fats in the bloodstream.

Cholesterol—(good) High-density lipoprotein (HDL) cholesterol.

Cholesterol—(dietary) Cholesterol present in food, especially in animal products.

Cholesterol—(bad) Low-density lipoprotein (LDL) cholesterol.

Coronary artery disease—Occurs when cholesterol plaque builds up (atherosclerosis) in the walls of the arteries to the heart.

Coronary artery spasm—A sudden vasoconstriction of a coronary artery depriving the myocardium of blood flow and oxygen. This may clinically manifest as chest pain referred to as variant angina or Printzmetal's angina.

Clotting factor—A substance in the blood that is needed for blood to harden and stop a wound from bleeding.

Collateral circulation—Compensatory circulation carried on through secondary channels after obstruction of the principal vessel supplying the part.

Computed tomography scanning—A technique for producing cross-sectional images of the body in which X-rays are passed through the body at different angles and analyzed by a computer; also called CT scanning or CAT scanning.

Congestive heart failure—Inability of the heart to efficiently pump blood through the body, causing buildup of blood in the veins and of other body fluids in tissue.

Coronary—Describes structures that encircle another structure, such as the coronary arteries, which circle the heart, and commonly used to refer to a coronary thrombosis or a heart attack .

Coronary arteries—The arteries that branch off from the aorta and supply oxygen-rich blood to the heart muscle.

Coronary artery bypass surgery—An operation in which a piece of vein or artery is used to bypass a blockage in a coronary artery; performed to prevent myocardial infarction and relieve angina pectoris.

Coronary heart disease—Disorders that restrict the blood supply to the heart, including atherosclerosis.

Coronary thrombosis—The blockage of a coronary artery by a blood clot.

# D

Dehiscence—A premature bursting open or splitting along natural or surgical suture lines. A complication of surgery that occurs, secondary to poor wound healing.

Defibrillation—A short electric shock to the chest to normalize an irregular heartbeat.

Diaphoresis—Perspiration; especially profuse perspiration.

Diuretic—A drug that increases the amount of water in the urine, removing excess water from the body, and is used in treating high blood pressure and fluid retention

Dyspnea—Difficulty breathing.

Dystonia—Disordered tonicity of muscle.

# E

ECG—EKG—An electrocardiogram; which is a record of the electrical impulses that trigger the heartbeat.

Electrocardiogram—An image of the heart that is created by high-frequency ultrasound sound waves.

Embolism—The blockage of a blood vessel by an embolus.

Endarterectomy—Surgery performed to remove the lining of an artery that has been narrowed by fatty tissue buildup.

Endemic—Describes a disease that is always present in a certain population of people.

Endocarditis—Inflammation of the inner lining of the heart, usually the heart valves; typically caused by an infection.

Endocardium—The inner lining of the heart.

Exercise stress test—The monitoring of the heart during strenuous exercise, usually on a treadmill or exercise bicycle, to evaluate how the heart responds to stress.

Exercise thallium test—An imaging test performed during and after an exercise stress test to evaluate functioning of the heart muscles.

Exogenous—Arising from outside of the body.

# F

Femoral artery—The main artery that supplies blood to the leg.

Fibrillation—Rapid, inefficient contraction of muscle fibers of the heart caused by disruption of nerve impulses.

# H

Hardening of the arteries—The common name for arteriosclerosis.

Heart attack—Myocardial infarction.

Heart block—A disorder of the heart caused by a blockage of the nerve impulses to the heart that regulate heartbeat.

Heartburn—A burning sensation experienced in the center of the chest up to the throat.

Heart failure—The inability of the heart to pump blood effectively through out the body.

Heart-lung machine—A machine that takes over the functions of the heart and lungs during certain types of surgery.

Heart rate—The rate at which the heart pumps blood, measured in the number of heartbeats per minute.

Heart transplantation—The transference of a heart from one human or animal to another.

Heart valves—Flaps of tissue that prevent regurgitation of blood from the ventricles to the atria or from the pulmonary arteries or aorta to the ventricles.

Heart valve prosthesis implantation—Surgical insertion of synthetic material to repair injured or diseased heart valves.

Hiatal hernia—A type of hernia, that occurs when a portion of the stomach protrudes through the diaphragm in the area where, the esophagus normally passes through.

Hiatus hernia—Protrusion of the stomach up into the opening normally occupied by the esophagus in the diaphragm, the muscle that separates the chest cavity from the abdomen.

Heart valve—The structure at each exit of the four chambers of the heart that allows blood to exit but not to flow back.

High-density lipoprotein—A type of protein found in the blood that removes cholesterol from tissues, protecting against heart disease.

Holter monitoring—A test which measures the heart rhythm (ECG) over a 24 hour period of time while the patient records their symptoms and activities in a diary. A small portable ECG device is worn in a pouch around the neck. After the test is complete, a correlation is made between the symptoms and activities recorded and the ECG pattern that was obtained simultaneously.

Hypercholesterolemia—An abnormally high level of cholesterol in the blood; which can be the result of an inherited disorder or a diet that is high in fat.

Hyperlipidemia—A general term for a group of disorders in which lipid levels in the blood are abnormally high, including hypercholesterolemia.

Hypertension—Abnormally high blood pressure, even when at rest.

# I

Infarction—Tissue death due to lack of blood supply.

Intensive care—Close monitoring of a patient who is seriously ill.

Intra-aortic balloon pump—A small balloon inserted into the aorta that helps to circulate blood by inflating between heartbeats.

Ischemia—A condition in which a tissue or organ does not receive a sufficient supply of blood.

# L

Lipid-lowering drugs—Drugs taken to lower the levels of specific fats called lipids in the blood in order to reduce the risk of narrowing of the arteries.

Low-density lipoprotein—A type of lipoprotein that is the major carrier of cholesterol in the blood, with high levels associated with narrowing of the arteries and heart disease.

# M

Mammary arteries—Arteries originating from the subclavian or axillary arteries and distributing to the anterior thoracic wall, mediastinal structures, diaphragm, pectoral muscles and mammary gland.

Magnetic resonance imaging (MRI)—A technique that uses magnetic fields and radio waves to create high-quality cross-sectional images of the body without using radiation.

Meniere's disease—A disorder of the inner ear, causing hearing loss, ringing in the ear, and the sensation that one's surroundings are spinning.

Mitral insufficiency—A problem with the ability of the mitral valve in the heart to close, which causes the heart to pump harder and reduces its efficiency.

Mitral stenosis—A condition in which the mitral valve in the heart becomes narrowed, making the heart work harder to pump blood.

Mitral valve—The valve in the heart that allows blood to flow from the left atrium to the left ventricle, but prevents blood from flowing back in.

Mitral valve prolapse—A common condition in which the mitral valve in the heart is deformed, causing blood to leak back across the valve; characterized by a heart murmur and sometimes chest pain and disturbed heart rhythm.

Murmur—A characteristic sound, that is heard through a stethoscope of blood flowing irregularly through the heart.

Myocardial infarction—The death of an area of heart muscle as a result of being deprived of its blood supply; characterized by severe pain in the chest; commonly called a heart attack.

Myocarditis—Inflammation of the heart muscle, which can be caused by a virus, and certain drugs, or radiation therapy.

Myocardium—The medical term for heart muscle.

# N

Night terrors—A form of nightmare causing abrupt awakening in terror; occurs mostly in children.

Nitrates—A group of drugs that widen blood vessels.

Numbness—The lack of sensation in a part of the body because of interruption of nerve impulses.

# O

Occlusion—The blocking of an opening or passageway in the body.

Open heart surgery—Any operation in which the heart is stopped temporarily and a machine is used to take over its function of pumping blood throughout the body.

Osteomyelitis—Inflammation of bone caused by a pyogenic organism. It may remain localized or may spread through the bone to involve the marrow, cortex, cancellous tissue and periosteum.

# P

Pacemaker—A small electronic device that is surgically implanted to stimulate the heart muscle to provide a normal heartbeat.

Pallor—Abnormally pale skin and usually refers to the skin of the face.

Palpation—The use of the hands to feel parts of the body to check for any abnormalities

Palpitation—An abnormally rapid and strong heartbeat.

Patent ductus arteriosus—A genetic disorder of the heart in which a channel connecting the pulmonary artery and the aorta fails to close and the heart must work harder to supply the body with blood.

Periarteritis nodosa—Inflammation and weakening of small and medium arteries

Pericardial window techniques—Surgical construction of an opening or window in the pericardium. It is often called subxiphoid pericardial window technique.

Pericarditis, tuberculous—Infection of the pericardium with tubercle bacilli. This condition arises by contiguous extension of tuberculous lesions of the hilar or mediastinal lymph nodes or by pleuropulmonary tuberculosis.

Pericardial effusion—Fluid buildup inside of the pericardium; affecting the performance of the heart.

Pericarditis—Inflammation of the membranous sac that covers the heart, causing chest pain and fever.

Pericardium—The membranous sac that covers the heart and the base of the blood vessels that are attached to the heart.

Peripheral vascular disease—The narrowing of blood vessels in the legs or arms, causing pain and possibly tissue death, as a result of a reduced flow of blood to areas supplied by the narrowed vessels.

Premature ventricular contraction—A cardiac arrhythmia which originates from within the ventricles. Isolated ventricular contractions are referred to as premature ventricular contractions.

Printzmetal's angina—A sudden vasoconstriction of a coronary artery; depriving the myocardium of blood flow and oxygen. This may clinically manifest as chest pain referred to as variant angina or Printzmetal's angina.

Pulmonary artery—The artery that supplies the lungs with blood from the heart.

Pulmonary edema—The buildup of fluid in lung tissue, which is usually caused by heart failure.

Pulmonary embolism—Blockage of the pulmonary artery by a floating mass in the blood.

Pulmonary fibrosis—A condition in which the tissue of the lungs has become thick and scarred, usually because of inflammation caused by lung conditions such as pneumonia or tuberculosis.

Pulmonary heart valve—The heart valve that stops blood pumped to the lungs from leaking back into the heart.

Pulmonary hypertension—Increased blood pressure in the arteries supplying blood to the lungs; caused by increased resistance to blood flow in the lungs, usually a result of a lung disease.

Pulmonary insufficiency—A rare defect in the pulmonary heart valve in which it fails to close properly after each muscle contraction, allowing blood to leak back into the heart; weakens the heart's pumping ability.

Pulmonary stenosis—Obstruction of the flow of blood from the heart to the lungs.

# R

Respiration—The process by which oxygen is taken in and used by tissues in the body and carbon dioxide is released.

Respirator—Another term for a ventilator.

Respiratory arrest—A condition in which a person suddenly stops breathing.

Respiratory distress syndrome—A condition experienced after an illness or injury damages the lungs, causing severe breathing difficulty and resulting in a life-threatening lack of oxygen in the blood.

Respiratory failure—The failure of the body to exchange gases properly, which leads to a buildup of carbon dioxide and a lack of oxygen in the blood.

Respiratory system—The organs that carry out the process of respiration.

Resting pulse—The pulse rate when a person is not experiencing any physical activity or mental stress.

# S

Saturated fat—Fats that contain the maximum amount of hydrogen possible, such as those found in meats and dairy products.

Septicemia—A life-threatening condition in which bacteria multiply in the blood and produce toxic materials.

Sinus bradycardia—A regular heart rate of less than 60 beats per minute.

Sinus rhythm—Normal heart rhythm.

Sinus tachycardia—A regular heart rate of over 100 beats per minute.

Sleep apnea—A condition in which breathing stops for very short periods of time during sleep.

Spasm—An involuntary muscle contraction; can sometimes be powerful and painful.

Staphylococci—Common bacteria that cause skin infections and a number of other disorders.

Stenosis—Narrowing of a body passageway.

Stent—A device used to hold tissues in place.

Stroke—Damage to part of the brain because of a lack of blood supply, and is due to a blockage in an artery, or the rupturing of a blood vessel.

Systolic pressure—The blood pressure measured while the heart is contracting.

# T

Tachycardia—A rapid heart rate of over 100 beats per minute.

Thallium stress test—This test is used to assess coronary blood flow before and after a period of strenuous exercise. Thallium testing involves the introduction of a radioactive tracer into the bloodstream. The radioactive tracer is then measured with a special camera and a determination of coronary artery blood flow can be made.

TPA—Tissue plasminogen activator or TPA is thrombolytic agent used to dissolve blood clots. TPA is introduced into a vein (intravenous) or directly into a blocked artery. Transient ischemic attack—A temporary block in the supply of blood to the brain, resulting in temporary loss of sensation, movement, vision, or speech; often called mini-strokes and can be precursors to a real stroke.

Tricuspid valve—The valve located between the two left chambers of the heart, the left atrium and the left ventricle.

Triglyceride—The main form of fat in the blood.

Carotid artery occlusive syndrome—Aortic arch syndrome, also referred to by many as vertebral-basilar artery disease.

# V

Valvotomy—Surgical correction of a narrowed heart valve.

Valvular heart disease—A heart valve defect.

Valvuloplasty—Reconstruction or repair of a narrowed heart valve.

Vascular occlusion—A sudden blockage of a blood vessel usually with a blood clot. Vascular patency—The condition of blood vessels, not being blocked or obstructed.

Vasoconstriction—Narrowing of blood vessels.

Vasodilation—Widening of blood vessels.

Vasovagal attack—A sudden slowing of the heart, causing fainting.

Vein—A blood vessel that carries blood toward the heart.

Ventilators-mechanical—Mechanical devices used to produce or assist pulmonary ventilation.

Ventricle—A small cavity or chamber.

Ventricular fibrillation—Rapid, irregular contractions of the heart.

Ventricular septal defect—A hole in the wall that separates the two lower chambers of the heart.

*Medical Glossary definitions supplied by American Medical Association Dictionary web site. (www.ama.org)*

www.ingramcontent.com/pod-product-compliance
Lightning Source LLC
Chambersburg PA
CBHW061335280526
45784CB00001B/22